The Portman Papers

LECTURES ON VIOLENCE, PERVERSION AND DELINQUENCY

The Portman Papers

LECTURES ON VIOLENCE, PERVERSION AND DELINQUENCY

Edited by
David Morgan and
Stanley Ruszczynski

Routledge
Taylor & Francis Group
LONDON AND NEW YORK

First published 2007 by
Karnac Books Ltd.

2 Park Square, Milton Park, Abingdon, Oxfordshire OX14 4RN
52 Vanderbilt Avenue, New York, NY 10017

Routledge is an imprint of the Taylor & Francis Group, an informa business

First issued in hardback 2019

British Library Cataloguing in Publication Data

A C.I.P. for this book is available from the British Library

ISBN-13: 978-1-85575-495-9 (pbk)
ISBN-13: 978-0-367-32531-2 (hbk)

Typeset by RefineCatch Limited, Bungay, Suffolk

CONTENTS

LIST OF CONTRIBUTORS

RICHARD DAVIES is a Consultant Adult Psychotherapist at the Portman Clinic and a former Director of the Clinic. He is a Member of the Psychoanalytic Section of the British Association of Psychotherapists and is in private practice. He is the editor of *Stress in Social Work* (Jessica Kingsley Publications, 1998) and the author of a number of journal articles and book chapters.

CARLOS FISHMAN is a Consultant Adult Psychotherapist at the Portman Clinic and the Clinic's Clinical Coordinator. He is a Fellow of the Institute of Psychoanalysis, a former Honorary Consultant at the London Clinic of Psychoanalysis and is in private practice.

AZ HAKEEM is a Consultant Psychiatrist in Psychotherapy at the Dartmouth Park Personality Disorder Clinic, Camden and Islington Mental Health and Social Care NHS Trust, and a Consultant Psychiatrist in Forensic Psychotherapy at the Portman Clinic. He is currently in training at the Institute of Group Analysis, London.

ANN HORNE is a former Consultant Child and Adolescent Psychotherapist at the Portman Clinic and is currently a Senior Honorary

Consultant at the Clinic. A Senior Member of the Child and Adolescent Section of the British Association of Psychotherapists, she is the joint editor (with Monica Lanyado) of *The Handbook of Child and Adolescent Psychotherapy* (Routledge, 1999) and *A Question of Technique* (Routledge, 2006) and the author of many journal papers and book chapters.

DOROTHY LLOYD-OWEN is a former Consultant Adult Psychotherapist at the Portman Clinic and is currently Senior Honorary Consultant at the Clinic. She is a Member of the Psychoanalytic Section of the British Association of Psychotherapists and is in private practice.

CARINE MINNE is a Consultant Psychiatrist in Forensic Psychotherapy at the Portman Clinic, Tavistock and Portman NHS Trust and at Broadmoor Hospital, West London Mental Health Trust. She is the Training Programme Director of the Specialist Registrar Training Scheme in Forensic Psychotherapy across these two Trusts. She is a Member of the Institute of Psychoanalysis.

DAVID MORGAN is a Consultant Adult Psychotherapist at the Portman Clinic and at the Chelsea and Westminster Hospital. He is a Fellow of the Institute of Psychoanalysis and is in private practice. He is the author of a number of journal articles and book chapters.

MARIANNE PARSONS is a Consultant Child and Adolescent Psychotherapist at the Portman Clinic. She is a Member of the Institute of Psychoanalysis, as both a child and adult psychoanalyst, and a Senior Member of the Child and Adolescent Section of the British Association of Psychotherapists and is in private practice. She is a former Head of Clinical Training at the Anna Freud Centre. She is the author of a number of journal papers and book chapters.

STANLEY RUSZCZYNSKI is the Clinical Director of the Portman Clinic and a Consultant Adult Psychotherapist at the Clinic. He is a Senior Member of the Psychoanalytic Section of the British Association of Psychotherapists and a Direct Member of the International Psychoanalytic Association and is in private practice. He has edited and co-edited four books (including *Psychoanalytic Psychotherapy in the Kleinian Tradition* [Karnac, 1999] and *Intrusiveness and Intimacy in the Couple* [Karnac, 1995]) and is the author of a number of book chapters and journal articles.

HEATHER WOOD is a Consultant Adult Psychotherapist at the Portman Clinic and is the Clinic's Research Lead. She is a Member of the Psychoanalytic Section of the British Association of Psychotherapists and is in private practice. She is the joint editor (together with Janice Hiller and Winifred Bolton) of *Sex, Mind and Emotion* (Karnac Books, 2006).

JOHN WOODS is a Consultant Child and Adolescent Psychotherapist at the Portman Clinic. He is a Senior Member of the Child and Adolescent Section and the Psychoanalytic Section of the British Association of Psychotherapists and a Member of the Institute of Group Analysis, and is in private practice. He is the author of *Boys Who have Abused* (Jessica Kingsley, 2003) and a number of book chapters and journal papers.

JESSICA YAKELEY is a Consultant Psychiatrist in Psychotherapy at the Portman Clinic and at University College Hospital. She is a Member of the Institute of Psychoanalysis and is in private practice.

INTRODUCTION

David Morgan and Stanley Ruszczynski

Actions speak louder than words. This statement is particularly true when we consider the effect that abuse, violence and perversion have on our society. The names Bulger, Dunblane, and Climbie immediately strike chords in our collective memories. In addition to these specific traumatic events we can add the ubiquitous news reports of abuses involving paedophilia, pornography and violence that occur in the world with remorseless frequency. And these are just the ones we hear about. Whether these abuses involve individual pathologies, or are the result of condoned acts in the name of political violence rather than expediency is an important distinction and beyond the scope of this book. However, the root causes and the end result of these actions are the same, that is, the destruction or corruption of the other in the interest of maintaining control or power.

Dr Mervyn Glasser, the eminent psychoanalyst, spent most of his career developing the Portman Clinic and wrote about the "core complex"(1979a, 1998). In this theory he described a mode of relating that avoided true intimacy. The subject, unable to bear a close relationship to the other due to claustrophobic anxieties involving fear of engulfment and loss of self through merger with the other, withdraws from intimacy in an attempt to control these fears. This retreat causes anxieties associated with agoraphobic fears of loss and abandonment leading to fears of disintegration. In an attempt to control these two extremes the subject endeavours to control the other so that engulfment and loss through too much intimacy or separation can be obviated. Behaviours that allow for continuing involvement with the other but eschew intimacy are employed. These behaviours always involve sado-masochism. They allow contact with the other but in specifically controlled situations dominated by violence, cruelty and pain. This can take the form of trans-generational relationships involving the enslavement and sexual abuse of the young; trans-sexuality, involving the manipulation of gender; fetishism, the idealization of substance over human involvement; exhibitionism, the projection of sexual anxieties into vulnerable onlookers; voyeurism, the reversal of paranoid fears through the secret observation of others; and various criminal activities which can be a means to reverse impoverishment and deprivation by attacking the life, sexuality or property of others as in murder, rape and theft. In all these situations it is the perpetrator that attempts to maintain equilibrium of their internal psychological world by creating fear, vulnerability and loss in the victim.

Sometimes the victim is an innocent bystander, unwittingly caught up in an unconscious enactment by others, or as in masochistic behaviour the victim is a willing accomplice, subjugating themselves to the other for core complex reasons. A recent example of the former was reported in the media, a violent attack by a man on a young woman in front of her young child. The victim of the attack survived despite the fact that the man clearly had murderous intentions toward her. This type of incident and other forms of physical or sexual assault often lead to intense speculation from various sources as to the cause and effect of such anti-social behaviour. Political representatives speak in clichés about the mentally ill, and members of the health, social and probationary services complain about serious lack of resources, both physical and emotional, with which to manage and provide treatment for offenders who may go on to act out their grievances on the minds and bodies of other people. Other factors cited are the closing of the big mental asylums and the neglect imposed upon our most vulnerable members of society by the so-called 'Care in the Community' policies. The latter is an apparently enlightened attitude towards the mentally ill leading to the closure of many large in-patient hospital settings. However, with prison populations now soaring it could seem that incarceration rather than containment and/or treatment has taken the place of the old hospital regimes.

This apparent disregard for the most vulnerable members of our society, and this includes both the perpetrator and the victim, lies at the heart of many of the disturbing headlines often to which we are exposed.

The first emotional response to most disturbing events is flight, to turn a blind eye. It is often too frightening and painful to think about what occurs in the minds of human beings who perpetrate these actions, and the effect it has on those whom it unwittingly involves. It challenges our own sense of security about the society we live in and our understanding of human behaviour. It might also make us uncomfortably aware of the thin line between those who enact sexual and/or violent crimes on the bodies and minds of others and those like ourselves who do not.

The second response is fight, to become angry and to want to inflict serious punishment on the perpetrators of these actions. The behaviours that impel us towards these powerful emotional responses include murder, paedophilia, rape, incest and complex sexual perversions. They create a sense of moral outrage in us that understandably makes us want to distance ourselves from these actions. There is no better way of doing this than to judge the perpetrator as inhuman and therefore to feel morally justified to exclude them from any reasonable thinking. Thus actions beget actions and all thinking can become subsumed into a knee-jerk reaction that puts the perpetrator of these crimes outside society. In this way thinking about the causes of these behaviours can be obviated, and action aimed at expelling the difficult and painful process that might lead to understanding, increased.

In this we can see our governments advocating tougher measures to tackle crime. Although sometimes presented as socially thoughtful, for example 'Tough on Crime Tough on the Causes of Crime', these seem more readily to espouse the tough punishment advocating action over thinking about cause. The latter can be seen as the worst kind of liberalism which all governments fear becoming associated with. As one recent prime minister put it, 'We should condemn a little more and understand a little less'. The problem with this approach is that if we meet pathological behaviours with only punitive action it merely confirms in the mind of the offender or abuser the condemnatory aspect within themselves, which is a cruel corrupt authority seeking power and control rather than understanding. This is an example of the core complex, these actions distancing the perpetrator from closeness and understanding and intimacy. This risks exacerbation of the behaviour rather than any possibility of change. Any change in the minds of those who live in cruel worlds may depend upon the experience of a mind in the other (a therapist) that is capable of meeting the mind of the perpetrator without becoming abusive or a victim.

If we return to the man who attacks a young woman with her child present, it could be seen to be reversing his own experience of abuse; feeling helpless in the face of a violent parental couple and emotional neglect and abuse from them, his childhood carers. In his murderous actions he unconsciously creates a situation where the victim's child observes the abuse and violence towards their own mother by a murderous man. This is the perpetrator, through a process of reversal, relieving himself of his own violent primal scene by evacuating it. This is an enactment at a physical level; he is not capable of using a mental mechanism such as projective identification to relieve his emotional pain, the pain having been triggered by seeing a caring mother–child couple. This is not an excuse to justify the man's actions but it might help to begin to understand what his actions reveal about his motivation. This does not help his immediate victim and she requires justice. However, just incarceration without containment and treatment, will not lay the beginnings of an understanding that he himself may at some time be capable of, and thus produce change in the way he deals with his past experiences and increased safety for society. This can also be used to educate us into preventative work with parents and children that might alleviate the risk of vulnerable people being left to enact their pain on others. A pre-emptive strike of thinking on those who live in worlds dominated by action might be the beginning of providing more sophisticated modes of communication other than physical concrete enactment.

Another traumatic example would be the apparently motiveless murder of Jamie Bolger by two young boys. This traumatized all of us. How can we explain these seemingly motiveless horrors? Again we can turn away and not think, build larger walls around children, restrict their movement, or we can go on witch hunts like the baying crowds outside the court where Jamie Bulger's young killers were tried: flight and fight reactions. If we consider the meaning of the boys' extreme actions we might see that what they communicate is not meaningless. A child abducted and killed a long way from anyone who could intervene and save him is a chilling enactment. This is surely the sad story of the two killers, whose emotional and psychological neglect and isolation in negative impoverished circumstances may have led to this enactment. This aspect of society is discussed in Shengold's book, *Soul Murder* (1989).

It is a dreadful irony and an appalling comment on our apparently civilised society that the two boys who perpetrated this crime have probably received better help and education than they would have done had they been left in their respective homes and environments. Prior to this caring and necessary state intervention they had been left, as a young man seen at the Portman following enactments but not murderous ones, so eloquently put it, to "write their story on the minds and bodies of their victims".

In a less dramatic but still violent way a woman writes her history on her unborn baby. She repeatedly becomes pregnant and is abandoned by unreliable boyfriends and comes into treatment following several abortions. During treatment she is shocked to discover that she has enacted her own early life experience. Her father, having impregnated her mother with her, abandoned the family to work abroad (ironically helping repatriate families.) She did not see him again until she was 12. Her concrete enactment is an attempt to gain mastery over an early experience; she creates a new life, the foetus, she becomes the mother, and the father is played by the abandoning boyfriends. The denouement is that the patient's own experience of abandonment has been enacted and projected into the now dead foetus. Welldon (1988) describes how women tend to enact their perversions towards their own bodies and/or their own children. This could suggest a suicidal wish towards oneself, a wish that one had never been born, perhaps stemming from the reality of this patient's early life and the ambivalence around her own birth. This patient's actions again exemplify the workings of the core complex; her attempts to develop intimate relations with a partner and their child are undermined by her ambivalence stemming from the experience of her own origins, being left with her depressed single mother, with its attendant fears of engulfment and merger and the distant abandonment by her father. It was a feature of this patient's early analysis that she frequently attempted to leave for work abroad with children, an attempt to leave her analyst holding the baby of the analysis when the developing analytic intimacy was becoming unbearable.

These cases demonstrate how after years of abuse and neglect the acted-on child, adolescent and adult eventually enact their own experiences by abusing and neglecting another. This reversal of their own experience is an attempt to evacuate into others their unbearable experiences. John Bowlby first drew attention to the connection between early attachment experiences and criminal behaviour. In his seminal paper '44 Juvenile Thieves' (Bowlby, 1944), he made the connection between anti-social tendencies and early experiences of prolonged separation. More recently Farrington (2003) provided corroboration showing that the best predictors of offending were early symptoms of hyperactivity, marital discord, harsh and erratic parenting and early experiences of separation from a parent. These experiences lead to insecure attachment.

We know that the capacity to feel deeply with another human being and for this feeling to be reciprocated, is one of the most profound experiences that any of us can expect, and this capacity for deep involvement with significant others depends on our earliest experiences. How I experience you and within that experience the emotional relationship we have, affects how I feel about myself, and my knowledge of myself reflects how I feel known by the other and consequently how I will treat others. If we are fortunate, one of the things we might get to know about ourselves is that our experience of our angry, envious and spoiling feelings leads to the capacity for cruelty and destruction. We all have this pleasure in destruction and it is our experiences in our early life that might help us to bear this aspect of ourselves and not be drawn into cruel and destructive actions. An excess of pleasure in human destructiveness seems to be in inverse proportion to the weakness of love of human commitment (Brenman 2003). There has often been little exposure to the power of a loving intercourse between parents or to warmly attuned care producing secure attachments to parents in the patients described in this book. They have been exposed to violence and corruption at the hands of their caretakers, violent couples and parental figures who appear to use their children as receptacles for their own psychosis or disturbance. These papers demonstrate the severe difficulties in working to help modify patients' behaviour, when the basic requirement for parental containment has been replaced by infants used as receptacles for experiences of violence and loss. The damaging early lives corrupt the individual, making it likely that they will turn from positive life and relationships to the refuge of cruelty in either its masochistic or sadistic form.

Over the many years of treating severely ill patients at the Portman Clinic clinicians have come up against silent deadly self-destructive forces in their patients which can seem antithetical to any help or change. These are patients in whom it seems the perverse pleasure of physical or emotional annihilation takes over from fear of loss or death. With these patients it is easy to undervalue the role of defensive life giving hate as a way of keeping something alive and which guards against fear of annihilation.

It is clearly important to develop an awareness of destructiveness in the treatment of these patients but it has to be balanced with the recognition of the victim reality of their profound trauma which often has complex trans-generational origins, that might only finally find expression in their complex destructive enactments. These may at first feel incoherent and mad.

The following are examples of apparent incoherence. A violent gangster was admitted to hospital because he was being driven mad by a persistent auditory hallucination of beautiful music emanating from radiators in his home. If it were communicated as a dream we might have been able to develop some mutual conscious understanding, but the problem here is experienced as a reality. We might understand that the gangster has placed his gentleness, his goodness, the longing for an idealised merged state with his mother, i.e., perhaps the music of his soul, into the radiator, a thing of warmth, and it is now persecuting him. The patient is locked in a world where there is no symbolic meaning. A transsexual man wants to cut off his 'old man' (his penis). When it is suggested to him that it might have something to do with his castrating father he feels attacked and threatened and describes his therapist as a "mind fucker". It seems that it is felt to be more violent to use his mind than mutilate his body. It seems the only person that might have any understanding in these cases is the therapist, but how does this understanding get communicated to patients living in such concrete worlds? By the very act of communication, however, there is somewhere the wish to be understood.

All the clinical work in this book shares the idea that one can repair damage to an internal object. The great disadvantage for our patients in this work, however, is that they often feel justified in their grievances. When working with perverse, psychotic or borderline patients, or criminal patients who enact their psychosis on the minds and bodies of others, for a great deal of the time one has to bear the experience of sharing one's mental space with someone whose communications can at first feel quite mad and may do so for some time. The papers in this book arrive as a result of experienced and courageous clinicians sitting with these patients, listening to them and suffering this experience, and this leads to understanding that has helped their patients. This is sometimes very difficult, not just because of our patients being disturbing, but also due to a social climate that is more likely to condemn rather than try to understand. All forensic settings can be used as receptacles to be projected into, and this can make it very difficult for the clinicians working in these settings to see their work as a valued achievement, tending to the sick and marginalized in our society. In the Portman Clinic we try to counteract this tendency in ourselves and in society by attending to our professional needs individually and as a group to process the effects of sharing our mental space with our patients' adverse experiences and actions.

It can often feel that there has been the introjection of an object performing the obverse of containment. Bion (1957) stressed the function of a containing object which is to make things thinkable, understandable and tolerable. He described the process of projective identification whereby a child can have a parent into whom they can project feelings, good and bad, for parental understanding. It is the parent who can name things and make sense of these sensations for the child, using their own experience of having been understood. To do this the parent must have the capacity to bear the psychic pain the child cannot tolerate. Repeated experience of this process leads to an internalisation of a thoughtful object which enables the child to deal gradually with anxiety and pain themselves.

When this process goes wrong the object is felt to be impervious to the child's projections. They are not acceptable and are returned unprocessed into the child and appear as a nameless dread. The child is used as a receptacle for the parents' return of the projections. This involves the introjection of an object, which is not only impervious but also overflowing with their own difficult projections, looking for a place to be understood and now residing in the mind of the infant. As the introjection of a good object is helpful in establishing links and organising a coherent structure, the introjection of an uncontaining object has the opposite effect, disrupting and fragmenting the development of personality (Williams 1998).

A patient who exemplified this was a concern to her parents because she was failing at school after having been previously successful. She had become increasingly withdrawn. She was referred after she had become violent towards a number of male teachers who had appeared to have formed good relationships with her at school. In the assessment she was able to talk to her male therapist about her parents sending her but then lapsed into a silent beseeching look which made the therapist feel extremely uncomfortable. Later, as this interaction was repeated endlessly the therapist felt trapped with this silent patient who had stopped talking. There was a feeling that something was being communicated accompanied by a worry that he was being incompetent. As each session came and went it added to the sense of cumulative dread and disappointment.

After six months of this behaviour, the patient responded to what was becoming a rather formulaic interpretation, that she was showing him what it felt like to be with someone who creates a feeling that something is about to happen, only to be disappointed, and how this might actually have been her experience or her fear of what might happen here. She then told him about sexual abuse by her father. The behaviour the therapist had been living through over the previous six months now seemed clearer. At one level the excitement with her father was addictive, but at another level it was unwanted, hated and out of her control. She seemed to need to enact this with the therapist, getting him excited about her possibly making a verbal communication and then leaving him disappointed and her in control. In some ways she had to see if he could bear it before she could put this experience into words.

The enactment continued because the situation was now reversed —and the therapist was now in the same position as she was. Should he remain silent as she had done or use the information she had given him in confidence? Her dilemma of when to speak or not now became his. Her father had left her with the confusing problem of what to do with adults who do not know the difference between hurting and taking care. As his daughter's sexuality had developed, her father had been unable to contain her ordinary projections about her sexual development into him and had used her by action as a container for his own pain and sadistic gratification. The question seemed to be how we help an adult who deals with their own muddle about their sexuality by putting it into their child and making them muddled about their own feelings.

Anna Freud (1965) felt that evil was reparable when she was working with the victims of the Second World War and that only love could mitigate hate. The whole therapeutic process is sustained by the belief that loving human and relational elements are the factors that modify cruelty. In sexual perversions there seems to be a distorted development of the entire personality and mental structure where sexualisation and violence become a mental state which is used to withdraw from reality and having to relate positively to the world. This withdrawal avoids any humanising influences.

So the problem in treating these patients is they feel that they have to resist the powerful forces of humanisation, love and concern, the importance of ethical thinking and truth, because these things we might consider to be positive life forces are the very things that are likely to make them aware of the paucity of their existence and stimulate envy. What we think is life giving may be perceived as an horrendous threat. Thus a patient told their therapist that if she believed in the truth of the therapy and that it met a real need in her, she feared she would become a feral child, unable to control herself, which would leave her with the choice of destroying the therapy by leaving or gorging herself on food until she killed herself with obesity. Thus she was terrified of her destructiveness towards the object but she was also aware that after such a length of time of neglect and cruelty both as victim and perpetrator, an awareness of something good and truthful would be too envy provoking and painful to contemplate.

André Green (1986) considers the destructive drive in these

patients to be aimed at destroying the meaning of everything that is good, good has to be rendered meaningless. Real destructiveness or what he terms evil is not the opposite of love, but an absence of it. This destructiveness is an attack on the emotions and the threatening awareness of any relationship between human objects which might make emotional life possible. These attacks are occasioned by a particular form of pleasure which makes destructiveness the preferred mode of enjoyment. It involves a desire to attack any knowledge and respect for understanding the basic need for human relationships. In its most primitive form, as seen in sado-masochistic patients at the Portman, it is the fascination of absolute destructiveness and domination of the helpless victim (as a projection of their own maltreated self) which gives rise to this pleasure.

The major reason for this book is not just to describe the effects of abuses on the minds of our patients or to catalogue in detail the crimes committed by them or against them. It is to highlight the role of the therapeutic worker who is often at the end of a transgenerational line of enactment. In this position we are being asked to bear the unbearable, the knowledge that we are being asked to know about can seem to be black holes in the psyche being passed down from one generation to the next. As Lanyado and Horne *et al.* (1999) state "it is the cumulative traumatisation that can take place within the worker's mind if we are not adequately supported that requires thought." One task of this book is to share the difficulties of this work and provide hope for those of us who can at times feel that we are working with hopeless cases. These patients, feeling like lost souls, can feel their only hope is to gain mastery over their experience by breaking the spirit of those who work with them. It is only by helping each other and sharing our experience of this difficulty that we can hope to bring light into this darkness. We hope this book is a contribution to this process.

The Portman Papers

LECTURES ON VIOLENCE, PERVERSION AND DELINQUENCY

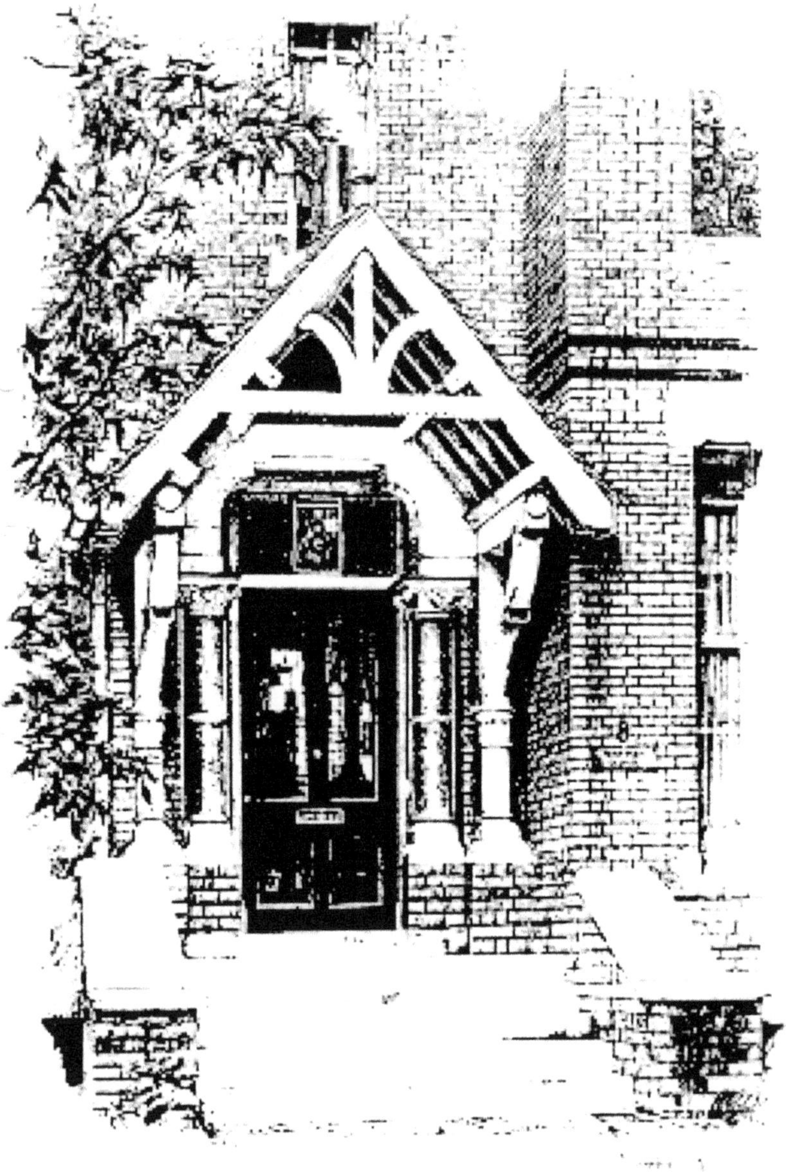

CHAPTER ONE

The Portman Clinic

An historical sketch

Carlos Fishman and Stanley Ruszczynski

The Portman Clinic began in 1931 as the Psychopathic Clinic and was the clinical arm of the Institute for the Scientific Treatment of Delinquency, later to be called The Institute for the Study and Treatment of Delinquency (ISTD) (Glover, 1960; Dicks, 1970). The Institute was founded by a small group of people impelled by the research of Dr Grace Pailthorpe, a psychiatrist and psychoanalyst, who had worked as a doctor in the trenches during the First World War. After the war she worked in Birmingham and Holloway Prisons. She became interested in the personality of women prisoners and wrote *Studies in the Psychology of Delinquency* (Pailthorpe, 1932). Her approach and her research attracted like-minded psychoanalysts including Edward Glover and Kate Friedlander, and their shared interests and, more importantly, Edward Glover's impetus and dedication, founded the Institute and with it the idea of developing a Clinic. Glover was already developing the understanding of sexual perversions, criminality, and addictions, and had also been Director of the London Clinic of Psychoanalysis.

Later, when writing about the beginnings of the Institute, Glover stressed that "The first concern of the ISTD (was) to make a *thorough examination* and the second to arrive at a *provisional diagnosis*. The diagnosis should be sound enough to permit of a satisfactory *recommendation of disposal;* the examination should be comprehensive enough not only to exclude diagnostic error but to permit of subsequent ... research" (Glover, 1960). So, from its very inception, the Portman Clinic had as its purpose assessment, treatment and research. In addition, Glover wrote that because delinquency and crime are social phenomena they appropriately attract the attention of a variety of disciplines including social workers and social psychologists. However, in his view, "... the most fundamental approach to crime, pathological or otherwise, is that of psychoanalysis" (Glover, 1960). This view remains central to the work of the Portman Clinic, which, whilst fully recognizing the necessary team work between the various disciplines involved in the care, treatment and containment of delinquent, perverse and violent patients, takes upon itself the task of refining and developing the in-depth understanding of the unconscious forces operating in the psychic make-up of its patients and of the patients of those professionals who approach the Clinic for consultation or teaching.

Perhaps it is not surprising that the Portman Clinic was born at a time in the history of the twentieth century that was particularly stormy. The period between the two great wars saw the birth of Communism, the rise of National Socialism and important developments in the move from fascism to democracy. Most of those who were associated with the early days of the Portman Clinic shared a particularly idealistic view influenced no doubt by the enthusiasm which Freud's theories of the mind encouraged in the early days. One can glean from documents that refer to the early days of the Clinic the belief that perhaps "*treatment*" might replace "*punishment*". Over seventy years later, and with the accumulation of substantial clinical experience, that idealism has certainly been modified and has evolved into something more realistic and therefore more hopeful. Portman clinicians treat individuals with complicated and severe psychopathologies using psychoanalytic psychotherapy, believing that, as Glover wrote, "... so long as the existence and power of unconscious motives is disregarded, we cannot learn any more about crime than an apparent commonsense dictates. ... However speculative and uncontrolled some psychoanalytic views on crime may be they do at least promise to uncover the fundamental flight from reality that leads to pathological and possibly all forms of criminal conduct" (Glover, 1960, p. xiii). This understanding of the disavowal of reality as being at the heart of much perverse, violent and delinquent behaviour sustains much contemporary clinical practice in the Portman Clinic today.

Early vice-presidents of the Institute for the Study and Treatment of Delinquency included Alfred Adler, Havelock Ellis, Sigmund Freud, Ernest Jones, Carl G. Jung, Emmanuel Miller, Otto Rank and H. G. Wells among others. One can see that the founding members of the Institute obtained the support of important intellectual figures of the time. As with many such ventures, funding was a major difficulty and apparently seeking charitable donations for the study and treatment of criminality was not easy, and there were serious struggles in this respect in the early days. It is very likely that support of such figures did help to secure some funding.

Dr Edward Glover was the main promoter of the Institute developing a clinical arm. The idea was that through a clinic the treatment aims of the institution would be complete. Initially, clinicians volunteered to see patients referred to them through the Clinic in their own consulting rooms and at much reduced fees so as to fulfil the charitable purposes of the Association. The Clinic saw its first formal patient on the 18th September 1933, "a woman, 47 years of age, noted as having a violent temper, charged with assault on her woman employer" (Saville & Rumney, 1992). At that time the staff of the Clinic included Dr Bion, Dr Eder, Dr Aubrey Lewis (one of the pioneers of psychiatry in the UK), Miss Barbara Low, Mr Adrian & Mrs Karen Stephen, Dr John Rickman, Mrs Melitta Schmideberg and others, many of them pioneers of psychoanalysis in Britain.

Later on, in the mid-thirties, the arrangement at the Clinic changed. With the help of Emmanuel Miller (the founding father of the first Child Guidance Clinic and an early supporter of the ISTD) the Clinic secured a room at the Western Hospital. The doctors, lay therapists, psychologists and social workers worked without payment. The clinic room was available mornings only. Five shillings had to be paid to the Western Hospital each time it was used. The physical examination was carried out by the hospital and psychometric examination by a psychologist on the Clinic staff. Where psychotherapy was necessary, it continued to take place in the therapist's own rooms.

The Institute for the Study and Treatment of Delinquency and the

Clinic found their first own home at number 8 Portman Street, London W1 in May 1937, and the Clinic centralized its services there starting in February of the following year. The present Portman Clinic carries its name after the street where it was first located, and replaced the earlier, rather contentious, name of "Psychopathic Clinic".

During the Second World War the staff of the Clinic was reduced considerably due to many joining the military. Despite the war clinical work continued, in a limited way: only assessments and short-term treatments were undertaken. Most of this was undertaken by a small group of psychiatric social workers that staffed the clinic during this time.

After the war the Clinic moved again, this time to Bourdon Street in Mayfair, and it seems that at the time the Clinic was located between a residence for nuns on one side and a brothel on the other! It was just before and after the war that many well-known psychiatrists and psychoanalysts, such as Dr John Bowlby, Dr Wilfred Bion, Dr William Gillespie and others, joined the staff of the Portman where they spent a part of their early psychiatric career.

With the coming into being of the National Health Service Act of 1948 the Clinic was formally separated from the ISTD and became part of the NHS. It was at this time that the Portman Clinic formally took its name, although it was still housed with its parent organization. After the Clinic joined the NHS a number of very creative developments occurred. Many of the staff who have contributed significantly to the literature of the psychoanalytic understanding of sexual perversions and delinquency gradually joined the Portman. Major works of Dr Glover and later Dr Glasser, Dr Limentani, Dr Weldon and others emanated from their work at the Portman. Classical papers of Edward Glover, contained in his book *The Roots of Crime* (1960), and also *The Early Development of Mind* (1956) were influenced directly by his work at the Portman. In the same vein, Mervin Glasser's seminal papers: "From the Analysis of a Transvestite" (Glasser 1979b), "Some Aspects of the Role of Aggression in the Perversions" (Glasser, 1979a) as well as "On Violence: A Preliminary Communication" (Glasser, 1998), were all based on his clinical work at the Portman Clinic. Adam Limentani's contributions included: "Clinical Types of Homosexuality" (Limentani, 1989c), and "A Re-evaluation of Acting Out in Relation to Working Through"

(Limentani, 1966). Estela Welldon's work on female perversion *Mother, Madonna, Whore* (Welldon, 1988) was also based on her clinical work at the Portman Clinic.

In 1961 the Portman Clinic organized a conference as a contribution to the celebration of the World Mental Health Year. This successful two-day conference resulted in the publication of the first edition of the well-known volume on the pathology and treatment of sexual deviation, *Sexual Deviation*, edited by Ismond Rosen (Rosen, 1964). This volume has seen two subsequent editions. The second edition (1979), probably the most widely quoted, includes a greater number of major contributions by the then staff of the Portman Clinic.

In 1970 the Portman Clinic moved to its present location in Fitzjohn's Avenue, London, a house adjacent to the Tavistock Centre. Together with the Tavistock Clinic it was at the time under the management of the Hampstead Health Authority. The Portman was a vibrant institution staffed, as always, along multi-disciplinary lines, having Clinical Psychologists and Psychiatric Social Workers, as well as Consultant Psychotherapists and a Consultant Physician. Most had trained as either psychotherapists or psychoanalysts. During the eighties a serious review of the role of psychotherapy was undertaken by the NHS and the special and dedicated work of those at the Portman Clinic and the Tavistock Clinic was organized under a special sub-committee of the Hampstead Health Authority. It was partly due to the standard of clinical work of both the Tavistock and Portman Clinics that the Seymour Report found that psychotherapy did have a continuing role to play in the NHS despite opposition (Seymour Report, 1985). Because of their standing as providing psychoanalytic psychotherapy services and training in the NHS, the Tavistock and Portman Clinics joined forces, and, as part of changes in the structure of the Health Services, the two jointly became an NHS Trust in 1994, and a Foundation Trust in 2006, whilst maintaining their separate identities.

During the late eighties, but principally during the beginning of the nineties a major change took place at the Portman Clinic. So far the staff had comprised doctors, psychologists and social workers, not all trained as psychoanalysts or psychoanalytic psychotherapists. In the late eighties the Portman Clinic was one of the first mental health institutions in the UK that created posts for non-medical adult psychotherapists and later on, in the early nineties and in recognition of the clinical work that non-medical staff did, all non-medical staff took the title of Adult Psychotherapists. Since then the clinical staff consists of Consultant Psychotherapists, Adult Psychotherapists and Child and Adolescent Psychotherapists and all are now trained as psychoanalytic psychotherapists or psychoanalysts.

The founding of the International Association for Forensic Psychotherapy was another of the major developments that the Portman Clinic was involved in during the nineties. This international organization was formed in recognition of the need for a dedicated forum for those psychotherapists that work with individuals suffering from criminality, sexual perversions and violence. Its origins lay in the European symposia where colleagues mainly from Holland, Belgium, Austria and Germany would meet with Portman staff to exchange views on the treatment of patients who had been involved with the criminal justice system because of their psychopathology. These symposia took place bi-annually, mainly under the leadership of Mervin Glasser, then Chairman of the Portman. Developing on these clinical exchanges Estela Welldon, a Consultant Psychiatrist, Psychotherapist and Group Analyst, who by then was already recognized internationally as an authority in the understanding of perversions in females, became the driving force behind the creation of the International Association of Forensic Psychotherapy. Since its founding, the IAFP has had ten international conferences in different parts of the world. Portman Clinic staff continue to play an important role in this association, contributing regularly to their international conferences.

It is perhaps because of the efforts of Estela Welldon and other members of staff of the Portman Clinic that the somewhat controversial title of Forensic Psychotherapist has come to exist.

Among many short conferences and courses initiated at the Portman Clinic for a variety of professionals in the mental health field, as well as the justice system, Mervin Glasser initiated a course on the Psychodynamic Understanding of Perversion and Delinquency. Estela Welldon then expanded this course into a two year, one day a week day release course for professionals working in the forensic field leading to a Diploma in Forensic Psychotherapeutic Studies. In addition, the Portman Clinic has been very involved, since very early in its history as a NHS institution, in the training of junior doctors who wanted to train as consultant psychotherapists. At present the Portman is involved in an imaginative arrangement with the educational authorities of the Royal College of Psychiatrists whereby junior doctors can do the double training as Forensic Psychiatrists and Psychotherapists, the forensic psychotherapy aspect of it being done at the Portman.

Finally, since being founded, the Portman Clinic has seen over twenty thousand patients and the substantial scientific contribution of the Clinic has been based on this clinical experience. A number of books and numerous papers and book chapters have emerged from the Clinic. We have referred to some above and many others will be referred to in the following chapters and in the bibliography. There is a further body of work to be edited as well as newly written, and published. This volume is the first of a series which will build on the work of our predecessors and further contribute to the psychoanalytic understanding of violence, perversion or delinquency.

CHAPTER TWO

The problem of certain psychic realities

Aggression and violence as perverse solutions

Stanley Ruszczynski

Introduction

Both Freud and Klein understood psychological development as grounded in the interweaving of love and hate, life and death instincts, involving both the body and the mind. In health, in the context of a benign parental environment, the normal development of the infant's instincts results in the strengthening of the life instincts and hence the lessening in the power of destructive impulses. The aggressive element of hate is contained, and comes under the influence of the capacity for concern for the other and therefore of love. Aggression may then be recruited in the service of passion and creativity and thus contribute towards the possibility of healthy relationships. As a result, true intimacy, which requires both the recognition of and respect for a separate other, becomes possible (Ruszczynski and Fisher, 1995). Sex, and in particular intercourse, is experienced as reparative and potentially creative, arousing little or no guilt.

However, this benign integration of physical sex and love is one of the most difficult achievements of human beings' psychic development. The full expression of intimacy, love and sexuality, requires the involvement of another and this dependence on another, an affront to narcissism and omnipotence, carries with it the inevitability of feelings of ambivalence towards that other. The achievement of this capacity for ambivalence, in reality a life-long struggle, is one crucial indicator of the potential for relatively healthy and mature relationships.

In the absence of this achievement of the capacity for ambivalence, love and concern do not temper and moderate aggressive instincts and aggression retains ascendancy. Fonagy has stressed the developmental need for normal aggression to be contained and writes that "violence is unlearned not learned". He says:

> models of aggression have tended to focus on how human aggression is *acquired*. Yet aggression appears to be there as a problem from early childhood, arguably from toddlerhood and perhaps from birth. Violence ultimately signals the *failure of normal developmental processes to deal with something that occurs naturally*.
>
> [Fonagy, 2003, p. 190, italics added]

In such circumstances relationships, sexual and non-sexual, are recruited in the service of malignant aggression, and sexuality in particular may be hijacked and become expressed as sadomasochistic, perverse and destructive. Robert Stoller refers to perversion as "the erotic form of hatred". He writes:

> Think of the perversions with which you are familiar: necrophilia, fetishism, rape, sex murder, sadism, masochism, voyeurism, paedophilia—and many more. In each is found—in gross form or hidden, but essential in the fantasy—hostility, revenge, triumph and a dehumanized object. Before even scratching the surface, we can see that someone harming someone else is a main feature in most of these conditions.
>
> [Stoller, 1976, p. 9]

Perversion

This understanding of the interlacing of sex and aggression, of love and hate, whether for loving or for malignant purposes involves both the body and the mind. It originates from Freud's delineation of mankind's "Oedipal destiny" (Hartocollis, 2001). Freud describes a 3- to 5-year-old boy's sexual attraction to his mother and his rivalry with and hatred of his father. He soon came to realise, however, that the young child pursues the love of the *opposite* sex parent with ambivalence because such a pursuit is feared to be at the expense of an affectionate attachment to the *same* sex parent. This dilemma is at the heart of the true nature of the triangular Oedipal situation, and hence feelings of ambivalence inevitably accompany any feelings of attachment, love or sexual expression.

Our Oedipal destiny is the inheritance of these conflicting libidinal and aggressive wishes, residing within the psyche from the beginning of life. Those who followed Freud, and especially those within the Kleinian tradition, postulate that the triangular Oedipal constellation is in fact confronted by infants from birth, because infants relate to their primary objects from birth, albeit in primitive ways. As such, libidinal and aggressive wishes are initially experienced in more absolute, narcissistic, fragmented and persecutory or idealized ways, inherent in the immature mind of the young infant, well before the classical Oedipus complex is reached.

Britton has elaborated an additional dimension to the Oedipal situation by highlighting that, as well as relating to the parents individually as mother and father, the young child, driven by natural curiosity, is confronted by the dim realization of a special link between the two parents, namely their sexual relationship (Britton, 1989). Children have to come to tolerate not only their exclusion from that special parental relationship, but also that the parental intercourse has a special quality because it may lead to the creation of a baby. Here is a highly charged and psychically demanding attack on the infant's omnipotence and narcissism.

The working through of the various elements of the Oedipal situation is parallel to what Kleinian writers refer to as the psychological development from the paranoid-schizoid to the depressive position. These positions refer to constellations of anxieties and defences that create particular states of mind and object relationships, the former more primitive and based on processes of splitting and projective identification and the latter resting more on a recognition of and concern for a valued and separate other.

To make this monumental developmental move the child has

to come to tolerate what Money-Kyrle refers to as the irreducibility of certain "facts of life", which have to be accommodated to, amongst which he includes dependence and the supreme creativity of parental intercourse (Money-Kyrle, 1971). Similarly, Chasseguet-Smirgel has described the need to come to terms with "the basic elements of human reality: the double difference between the sexes and the generations" (Chasseguet-Smirgel, 1985). She has suggested that failure to do so results in a regression to an "anal universe", where separateness and difference is disavowed. Segal too suggests the building of a "faecal empire" as a defence against separation (Segal, 1972). The language used by these writers, "human reality", "facts of life", and references to the defensive re-assertion of anality, suggests the fundamental necessity of coming to tolerate the anxieties and hatred caused by this loss of narcissism and omnipotence when confronted with difference and separateness.

Developmental difficulties might emerge at the threshold between the more primitive, narcissistic states of mind and the more mature depressive position. At this borderland, libidinal and aggressive instincts and hence the expression of love and hate, life and death forces, come into problematic conflict. If the loss of narcissism and omnipotence feels intolerable, if the capacity for ambivalence cannot be achieved, if hate retains an ascendancy over love, then aggression, violence and the disavowal or perversion of painful realities are likely to emerge as predominant expressions of emotional states.

Freud initially understood perversions as residues of infantile component drives that had not been sublimated. In his *Three Essays on Sexuality* Freud (1905) describes as perverse the regular intrusion into the adult's sexual life of the normal polymorphously perverse sexual and aggressive instincts of childhood. These partial instincts make up aspects of the ordinary and appropriate sexuality of children; some such behaviour may be contained in adult fantasies and in the foreplay of some peoples' ordinary sexual lives. What significantly differentiates such activity from a perversion is that perverse activity is compulsive, fixed, driven by hatred not love for the object and does not usually culminate in heterosexual intercourse leading to orgasm.

Though it is tempting to think that sexual perversions are primarily sexual and driven by sexuality, they are better understood as activities that *hijack* sexuality (Caper, 1999), recruiting it to accomplish ends that are fundamentally aggressive and destructive, resulting in what Stoller calls "eroticized hatred". The subject or patient themselves is also a victim of this violence and hostility, certainly in their mind and sometimes in their physical body, though this will often be overshadowed by the fate of their victim.

A significant development took place in Freud's understanding of perversion when he recognized the significant defensive functions of perversion, defending primarily against knowledge of aspects of the Oedipus complex (Freud, 1919, 1927). We would now say that what is perverted is knowledge of reality, both internal and external. This hatred of and attack on reality is likely to be a product of both the narcissistic and omnipotent aspects of the patient's personality and a defensive reaction to the unbearableness of the pain, humiliation and subsequent murderousness likely to have been experienced in their upbringing. The successful disavowal of reality requires sadistic control of the object and a splitting of the ego, creating an unconscious object relationship based on control and misrepresentation. Hence such relating is primarily sado-masochistic, perverse and based on corruption of truth.

In working clinically with perverse and violent patients, couples and individuals, I have come to find it useful to hold in mind the idea of *violation* as a central element in the sado-masochistic and violent act. It is essential to think not only about disturbed and disturbing violent or perverse behaviour, but also about a *perverse organization of the mind*, based on a particular constellation of anxieties, defences and internal object relations, which will get projected into the external world in a variety of ways (Ruszczynski, 2003). The violent act violates the other's body and their mind; the sexually perverse act is also likely to violate the other's body but the overriding central dynamic in the perverse act is the corruption of the other's mind by corrupting truth and reality, albeit often by sexual and aggressive means. I will say more about this later.

The Core Complex

Glasser (1979a, 1998) holds the view that central to the understanding of a perverse psychic structure is a dynamic psychic organization, which he calls "the core complex", in which aggression is an integral feature. The core complex has two elements and is a normal phase of development through which the infant has to pass. It describes the constant movement between the deep-seated longing for the most intimate closeness with the object, usually understood to be the mother—closeness to the degree of merger or union—and then a terrified flight away from this object because the desired merger threatens to result in the annihilation of the self.

Glasser goes on to suggest that this threat of annihilation may be dealt with in either of two ways. One way is a defensive narcissistic withdrawal. This is likely, however, to produce a sense of desolate isolation and abandonment, leaving only the self (both body and mind) as the focus for the aggression initially directed at the object. This may lead to a profound level of depression. Alternatively, the threat of annihilation by the engulfing object may provoke intense self-preservative aggression, acted out or in the mind, which, whilst aimed at securing the survival of the self, involves the destruction of the object, usually considered to be mother. Often, it is this aggression, if acted out, which brings the patient to the attention of the authorities or alerts the patient themselves to the dangerousness of their fantasies and impulses.

Both the narcissistic withdrawal and the aggressive attack on the primary object produce, in fantasy, the loss of the desired object and the terror of abandonment. This propels the patient back towards a desperate search for closeness and merger with the object and fear of engulfment may then re-emerge. Here we have the psychically disturbing circular nature of the core complex.

Henri Rey (1994) describes a similar psychic structure when he refers to the "claustro-agoraphobic" dilemma, which leaves the patient feeling that a place of safety and security cannot be found. Closeness to the desired object results in feelings of intrusion and claustrophobia, separateness from the object results in feelings of abandonment and agoraphobia. Similarly, Lewin and Schulz (1992) refer to the core pathology of the borderline patient as the "double danger of losing or fusing".

Such anxieties about engulfment and abandonment arise from the more infantile and primitive aspects of the personality, which appear to dominate the adult mind. We are referring, therefore, to an underlying psychotic structure with narcissistic and omnipotent features, and a preponderance of primitive or psychotic anxieties, defences and object relations. Intrusion into and mastery over the object is more likely than a capacity for concern or intimacy. Corruption of reality to meet narcissistically driven needs is equally more likely than a toleration of dependence, separateness, loss and ambivalence.

Faced with these overwhelming primitive anxieties, an attempt might be made to defend against them by *sexualization*: the defensive manoeuvres of narcissistic withdrawal or self-preservative aggression become eroticized. *This sexualization defends against the anxiety of the loss of the self or the other by creating the fantasy that rather than engulfment or abandonment there is an interpersonal object relationship.*

The sexualization of aggression results in masochism or sadism. When there has been a narcissistic withdrawal, only the self is available to receive the aggression initially directed at the threatening object. When this aggression directed at the self is sexualized, it leads to masochism. The masochist has a sense of control over the degree of suffering that will take place; there may also be a fantasy of control over the threatened abandonment and the feared annihilation. In addition, the masochist may feel that he is clearly not being aggressive to the object, who is therefore safe from his destructiveness. Unconsciously, the masochist also experiences the suffering as punishment, allaying some of the guilt for the aggression felt towards the object.

> A masochist man, who uses a dominatrix to torture and humiliate him, some time into treatment, is beginning to let himself know of his terrifying sense of emptiness, loneliness and resultant feeling of unworthiness. The pain and punishment he receives from the dominatrix temporarily relieves him of these feelings because with her he is the architect, not the victim, of his suffering and humiliation. By eroticizing the pain and abuse he gains pleasure from the experience as well as from the fact that he now has ultimate control over what is done to him. He behaves in a highly dangerous manner so as to omnipotently defy humiliation, suffering and terror, living out a fantasy that he can not only control but also ultimately survive and overcome the abusing hateful internal object, whose victim he felt himself to be. This is all in the service of gaining some sense of triumph and mastery over otherwise unbearable feelings and fantasies. This particular patient is also unconsciously punishing himself for having failed to rescue his mother from her depression and pain.

The sexualizing of self-preservative aggression, on the other hand, results in sadism, a wish to hurt and to control. In fantasy this preserves the object, which is now no longer threatened with destruction but is engaged with, albeit sadistically. It is not unusual to see this in couple relationships where one or both partners treat the other with hatred and contempt but cannot separate.

The sexualization, masochistic or sadistic, acts like a binding force, organizing and securing the object relationship. Sadistic and masochistic relating are ways of engaging intensively with another so as to militate against the dangers of separateness, loss, loneliness, hurt and destruction. Excited, intense feelings and experiences are used as substitutes for love and care. The excited eroticized repetition serves to defend against destructiveness, both one's own and that of the other. There is pretence that it is a kind of loving relatedness, an exciting exchange sought by both parties.

The differentiation between self-preservative aggression and sadomasochism is important in understanding the difference between the object-relating of the perverse patient and the violent patient. The differentiating factor is the attitude to the object at the time at which the act is carried out (Glasser, 1979a, 1998). In the *self-preservative aggressive* act, the destruction of the object is essential and its purpose is to eliminate the other who is perceived as life threatening. The object's emotional reaction, the meaning of the behaviour to the object, is irrelevant. The violent act is, in fantasy, life preserving. It seeks psychic equilibrium. This is a violent and cruel state of mind, and at the extreme is murderous. The *sadistic* act, on the other hand, seeks to torment and control the feared other whose emotional reaction is crucial: the specific aim is to cause the object to suffer, physically or mentally. As sadomasochism is based on this control and domination of the other, it requires *some*, albeit primitive, capacity to imagine the other's state of mind.

These states that I have described are, of course, never as clear cut in reality. Domination and control are essential features in both aggression and sadism. In self-preservative aggression they are sought only to negate the danger whilst in sadism they play a central role in entrapping and engaging the object. Let me give two clinical vignettes as illustrations.

A young female patient was referred for depression but also because she often found herself in disturbing sado-masochistic relationships. She had been raped on at least three separate occasions during her adolescence and early adult life. As a child she had been abused, emotionally and physically, first by her father and then, after being taken into care, by two sets of foster parents. She presented as generous and self-effacing, willing to put herself out for anyone, friend, neighbour or stranger. Her masochism, however, was barely hidden behind this pseudo-caretaker role and as treatment started it soon became clear how she ignored obvious signals of danger, often placing herself in positions where she could be manipulated, abused or raped. She often missed sessions and complained that I was not offering her times that she could manage. In the transference I became the inconsiderate and uncaring object and she the suffering victim. When she did attend, she would often say that it was for my benefit and not hers. Her partner abused her emotionally and, in effect, raped her for his sexual satisfaction. She masochistically sustained their relationship in the face of obviously cruel and violent treatment and triumphantly told me how she was prepared to survive his abusive behaviour because, she said, she had never felt as loved by anyone as she did by him. In the clinical work we came to see that in this masochism there was, in fantasy, a secret triumph over hurt, neglect and abuse. But to sustain this illusion of control and domination over her situation, she had to deceive herself about the degree of abuse she suffered. She corrupted the reality of being used and abused into a fantasy of "being loved". Occasionally, this perverse structure broke down and she became physically ill. Briefly, she would then feel murderous fury at her partner who continued to pay her no attention and persisted in demanding that she meet his requirements. Unconsciously terrified that her murderousness would destroy her object, she would rapidly reconstruct the masochism and re-establish her benign view of the relationship and, in the process, split off and evacuate her own feared aggression. To do otherwise would require her to face the pain and rage at the multiple losses, betrayals and abuses that she had experienced and which fundamentally threatened her sense of psychic and bodily survival. In the transference I became the abusing object seen as "forcing her" to think about her internal world and the ways in which she dealt with it.

A homosexual paedophile patient, who used young homosexual male prostitutes, started off his contact with a new prostitute in a mutually consensual, sado-masochistic relationship—with him taking the overtly masochistic role. Initially, he believed that this encounter would turn into a mutually loving relationship and that this might eventually help the prostitute to develop a better life, a manic and omnipotent idea that revealed the primitive nature of his thinking. When the prostitute inevitably let him down, my patient began to fear losing him. Initially his masochism increased, often at great personal cost, psychical and financial, in an attempt to secure the relationship. When this inevitably failed to secure the continued interest of the prostitute, my patient found himself having extremely sadistic and violent fantasies. It was his anxiety about acting on these fantasies, together with a growing sense of oscillating between this sense of murderousness and suicidal despair, which eventually led him to seek treatment.

As is implicit in both of these brief clinical vignettes, *there is always deception involved in masochism*—a secret contempt and desire to control is hidden behind the appearance of humiliation and submission. *Beneath masochism there is always an unconscious fantasy of omnipotent mastery over the feared and hated object, and the masochistic sexualization of the fear and hatred results in perceived pleasurable gratification from the suffering*. A masochist is therefore always at the same time a sadist, even though either the active or passive aspect may be the more strongly developed and represent the predominant activity.

The facts of life

Since sado-masochism is understood to be such a central feature of all perverse activities, we are led to the conclusion that there is always deception, misrepresentation and an attack on reality in the perverse act. And, because the perverse mental structure involves the whole personality, *the attack on or misrepresentation of reality is a fundamental and central feature of the perverse patient's psychic make-up.*

A female patient, multiply abused and violated in her childhood and adolescence, who now gets herself sexually abused by picking up men in the street and parks or sex clubs, said to me recently, "I can't stop doing this because I would then have to know what I was doing." She often refers to herself by a different name when she describes her very dangerous and perverse activities and says that she does not know this person who engages in these frightening masochistic behaviours.

Clinical perversion may therefore be understood as fundamentally defensive, achieved primarily by deception and disavowal of reality, with the purpose of fending off unbearable affects that would otherwise have to be known and experienced. Perverse phenomena could be described as deriving from destructive forces directed primarily against perception, both the perceiving self and the other who might prompt these perceptions. Perverse patients might therefore be described as unconsciously determined to pervert the capacities for thought and perception, not only their own but also those of people around them, including, of course, clinicians and other carers (Feldman, 2000).

A number of writers have paid particular attention to the understanding of perversion as the product of distortion and misrepresentation of reality. They stress, in particular, the disavowal of the reality of *the difference between the sexes and between the generations* (McDougall, 1972; Chasseguet-Smirgel, 1981, 1985; Steiner, 1993). For example, the paedophile denies the reality of the differences between adults and children, and, in doing so, denies one of the fundamental facts of life, that of the difference between generations. The transvestite may need to diminish or obliterate the reality of the difference between male and female.

One transvestite patient describes how successfully, in his view, he divides his life between his male-self and his female presentation. When cross-dressed, he thinks of himself as a woman and acts out various scenarios as if, in his perception, he is a woman. When not cross-dressed he leads an ordinary life as a man: he is married with children, has a sexual relationship with his wife and is professionally successful. He considers himself to have complete mastery over whether he is a man or a woman. He can be both, he says, with whichever gender role he is dressed up in being the gender that he considers himself to be. Though he talks of the differences between the two genders, we have begun to understand that actually he denies that any differences really exist. In his mind the differences are spurious or marginal—really there are no differences and he can transcend what there are at will. What is emerging in the clinical work is the view that there is a gulf between the genders such that each

> constitutes a separate universe, which cannot possibly be bridged. This seems to imply a very disturbed image of the internal couple—a fused and undifferentiated couple or a couple who are completely unknowable to each other. Either way there seems little possibility of the couple relating to each other. This has rather pessimistic therapeutic implications for the possibility of this patient even beginning to integrate the different aspects of himself in a more realistic way.

Misrepresentation of reality is central to an understanding of the perversions and arises from a specific mechanism in which contradictory versions of reality are allowed to coexist simultaneously. Freud initiated this understanding of the coexistence of competing realities, in his study of fetishism (Freud, 1927), but the mechanism described is applicable more broadly (Steiner, 1993). Freud says that the young boy assumes that there is no difference between the sexes. After the child is confronted with his observations of the reality of the differences between the genders, he may accommodate his powerful assumption of no difference by simultaneously holding the belief that his mother *does* have a penis whilst retaining his knowledge that she *does not*. The fetish is a substitute for the mother's penis that the little boy believed she had, a belief he does not want to give up, even when faced with material reality, because it raises castration anxieties: his anxiety that he too might suffer a similar fate and lose his penis. This holding on to contradictory beliefs is achieved by what Freud calls, "a rift in the ego, which never heals but increases as time goes on. The two contrary reactions to the conflict persist as a centre-point of a splitting of the ego" (Freud, 1940). Chasseguet-Smirgel suggests that this splitting be considered as a vertical split in the ego, with the perverse disavowal of reality existing *alongside* the recognition of reality (Chasseguet-Smirgel, 1985).

Money-Kyrle's delineation of three fundamental facts of life may be helpful to further our understanding of this perverse relationship to reality (Steiner, 1993). These are, "the recognition of the breast as a supremely good object, the recognition of the parents' intercourse as a supremely creative act, and the recognition of the inevitability of time and ultimately death" (Money-Kyrle, 1971).

The first fact, that the source of goodness required for the infant's initial survival comes from outside him (usually from mother), challenges omnipotence and narcissism and requires the toleration of separateness, dependence and gratitude. In the paranoid schizoid position, mechanisms of splitting and projective identification make possible illusions of omnipotence and narcissistic self-sufficiency. In the course of development there begins to be some integration of this omnipotent wish for self-sufficiency with the painful realization of attachment and dependence. However, this realization of separateness and dependence might feel too threatening and a defensive perverse structure may be created to accommodate a partial acceptance of the reality of separateness, difference and dependence but co-existing with a continued belief in omnipotence and self-sufficiency, with the latter retaining a primacy.

Aspects of this disavowal of separateness and dependence are often part of the psychic structure of abusive and violent marriages. In such marriages there appears to be a relationship between two separate people, but actually one, or usually both partners, are relating narcissistically, whereby, as a result of projective identification, the other person is actually seen as little more than an extension of the self. This is a perverse relationship because the partner's separateness is disavowed and they are in effect colonized and related to parasitically. When this colonization is felt to be challenged by the partners' ordinary independent behaviour, it might feel very threatening to the narcissist because it requires a toleration of separateness and dependence and hence a loss of omnipotence and narcissism. If this is felt to be intolerable, violent reactions might follow which are both an expression of the threat to the narcissistic self and a means of trying to recapture and control the other. Aggression and sadomasochism emerge as ways of dealing with the reaction to, and fear of, separateness and dependence.

The second fundamental fact of life described by Money-Kyrle is that of the true reality of the Oedipal situation. This involves firstly, tolerating knowledge of the parents' sexual relationship and tolerating being excluded from it; secondly, tolerating the generational differences between adults and children; and thirdly, recognizing the differences between the sexes which includes coming to know that babies come from heterosexual intercourse.

The reality of these facts of life can be denied by the solutions offered by some of the sexual perversions: these can be thought of as attacks on separateness, difference and the procreativity of the parental couple which cannot be tolerated. For example, the difference between the generations is denied in paedophilia and child sexual abuse. Homosexual intercourse might be understood in the clinical situation as an attempt to deny the differences between the sexes and to deny that new life is the product of the intercourse of these two sexes. Transvestism might be thought of as an attack on sexual difference.

> A transvestite patient states with total conviction that, when cross-dressed, he believes himself to be a women. He recently described the very specific way in which he holds his penis when masturbating thereby simulating, he thinks, a woman masturbating using her clitoris. When cross-dressed he straps his genitals in such a manner that they are in effect, forced back into his body, demonstrating his abhorrence of his penis and his attempt to eradicate the reality of its existence.

The third of Money-Kyrle's facts of life relates to the realities of passing time, of loss in its multiple forms and ultimately death. Facing and mourning losses, a constant necessity throughout life, is part of the reality of life that may feel so unbearable that loss is disavowed. This is connected with the pain of recognizing that from the beginning of life all good things have to come to an end, starting with the fact that access to the breast cannot go on forever. This makes us aware of the reality of its existence in the external world outside of our control (Steiner, 1993) and is an affront to any notions of our omnipotence and narcissism.

Sohn has suggested that some extremely dangerous and violent patients may be understood partially in relation to their experience of loss. He describes how their condition may be the result of a developmental history punctuated by a profound series of losses and a failure in the development of the capacity for symbolization (Sohn, 1997). For such patients "loss has been totally and psychotically denied", resulting in a psychological condition "in which total intolerance for any depressive experience leads to a need to act out physically" (Sohn, 1997). Hyatt Williams too suggests that a state of murderousness is derived from a failure to work through emotional disturbances engendered by experiences, thoughts, feelings and fantasies to do with loss, life threatening situations and death (Hyatt Williams, 1995).

I am reminded of one patient who was often preoccupied by cruel and murderous fantasies, especially when stimulated by news reports of brutal attacks, sexual abuse, killings or other such horrors. He was regularly involved in physically aggressive and violent encounters in his relationships and with near strangers, believing that this was the only way he could manage himself, his experiences and other people.

He began to be confronted by a sense of loss and endings, as a result of our addressing the beginnings and endings of sessions, holidays and other breaks in the treatment, transitions in the therapeutic relationship that he found almost intolerable. Initially, he oscillated between despair and rage at me: he said that I had "invented" time, and forced him to realize that he was neither omnipotent nor immortal, that time does pass on, that things do come to an end and that he cannot control any of it. His fragile and defensive narcissism had previously allowed for an illusory sense of timelessness and a fantasy of immortality so that losses need never be confronted and mourned. When he could not avoid awareness of loss he found himself getting involved in physical fights, often coming out the loser but feeling in some way cleansed by the experience. In addition, throughout his adult life he had had a serious of completely unnecessary facial cosmetic operations in the attempt to maintain his perceived youthful appearance. When we eventually discussed this, his terror at the idea of loss, including the loss of his own youth through the natural process of aging, was experienced as if a life and death matter. The loss of his youth was closely attached to an idea of him having "blemishes", which in his mind explained why he had been consistently rejected, abused and discarded in his childhood. This impossibly persecuting standard of perfection was also applied to his objects and came to be understood as a desperate defence against the extremely imperfect objects who had deserted him (his father died when he was one) and abused him (his mother emotionally and his aunt and subsequent carers sexually). Later in the treatment, when the reality of loss, including the passing of time and aging began to be more tolerable, he became shocked by his propensity for violence and by the medical assault he had perpetrated on himself. We slowly came to see that he had turned to both sadistic and masochistic aggression and violence to sustain a sense of triumph over the unacceptable losses and ravages of time and the physical and emotional blemishes that this inevitably produced. This had also helped him fend off the murderous hatred of his imperfect objects who, in their attitude and behaviour towards him, had defined him as imperfect, to be discarded or abused.

Perhaps in a less dramatic way, promiscuity might be one sexualized attempt to deny the passing of time when a constant seeking of new sexual conquests is used as a false reassurance to counter the realities of passing time, of aging and its attendant losses, ultimately death. Resorting to the timelessness of fantasy, be it romantic or base, might be another way to deny and overcome this fact of life. The narcissism and omnipotence that is severely threatened by this psychic reality might be further bolstered through fantasies of timelessness and immortality. It is only with the acceptance of time passing that time itself becomes a factor in patients' lives. Losses may then become more tolerable.

In his paper on fetishism (Freud, 1927), Freud refers to two patients both of whom were unable to face the loss of their fathers through their premature death.

> I am reminded of a late adolescent patient, referred for assessment and treatment following an indecent exposure and other sexual offences. He told me that he had talked to his father about the incidents which he now felt he understood. I knew, as did he, that his father had left him and his mother about 14 years previously, when the patient was about 3 years old, and that he had not seen him since. Given that he had this relationship with his father, the patient told me, there really was no reason to discuss the offences with me, especially as his father completely understood him, as I obviously did not.
>
> Another patient, who had violent fantasies about capturing, torturing and mutilating women talked at some length, in his assessment, about his relationship with his father. It was only when I, in passing, made some reference to his contact with his father that the patient then told me that his father had died nearly 30 years ago when he was 6 years old.
>
> Both of these patients found themselves having sadistic fantasies towards women and the first patient was beginning to enact these. Both spoke of profound difficulties in their current sexual relationships and described women as desired but also profoundly feared and experienced as intrusive and overwhelming.

Glasser has written that,

> what offers a different solution to those found by the pervert and the psychotic is . . . the presence of the father. With the father present,

> the infant can seek a solution to the core complex's "irreconcilable conflict of opposites" by turning to the father as an alternative object.
> [Glasser, 1985, p. 409]

I wonder whether the inability of these two patients to tolerate and accept their father's death prevented both of them from successfully completing the mourning process. It was as if each felt their father to be present though they both also knew, because they were not psychotic, that he was actually long absent or dead. If they had been able to tolerate their losses and mourn, it might have enabled them to integrate the father as an internal figure. He could then have been made use of intrapsychically as required when managing the core complex oscillation between abandonment and annihilation in relation to the mother.

Violence and sadism as perverse solutions

Perverse beliefs, sado-masochism and violence are turned to defensively when ordinary psychological development inevitably moves the patient towards having to recognize, tolerate and integrate these facts of dependence, Oedipal realities and the inevitability of loss. If these psychic realities are felt to be unbearable, perverse activities are enacted and perverse beliefs are developed both to suppress the knowledge of these realities and also to corrupt the mind's capacities to perceive and tolerate them. Simultaneously, the disavowal of certain facts of life, for example the significance of generational differences, legitimizes some sexual perversions and acts of violence. Denial and aggression are turned directly against the mind of the patient and through projective processes against the mind of his or her objects. Developmentally this locates such patients at the border of the paranoid-schizoid level of functioning.

Some patients act out perverse solutions in grossly perverse or violent acts. Others do not, but their states of mind and object relationships will be heavily influenced by perverse solutions. There appears to be no agreement as to the difference between those patients who actually act out their fantasies and those who do not, but it is very probable that destructiveness in the character is crucial in the perverse personality. Whether this excessive destructiveness is constitutional or whether it is the result of parental and/or environmental deprivation is open to debate and discussion. Probably both are present.

The crucial difference between those patients who actually act out their violence and perversion and those who do not might be related to a failure in infantile containment (Bion, 1962a). This would lead to a failure in the capacity to achieve some depressive position functioning and a failure in the capacity for symbolization (Sohn, 1997). Some patients turn their perverse solutions into fantasies or dreams, but others have no capacity for such mentalization and so have to act them out.

Hyatt Williams and Sohn, amongst others, have suggested that enactments of aggression, violence and murderousness are induced by the psychic toxicity resulting from certain emotional experiences being unprocessed as a result of a failure or lack of containment (Hyatt Williams, 1998; Sohn, 1997). Fonagy and Target (1995) assert that violence is a product of the person's lack of a capacity for reflection or mentalization. Without the experience of containment, no development of a psychological self can take place, a self that can process and think about experiences and psychic states. This cannot happen because such development requires the primary experience and perception of oneself, in another person's mind, as thinking and feeling. Fonagy and others make this point powerfully when they write that, "Freud, arguably, saw infancy as a time when the self saw others as extensions of itself ... our emphasis is the reverse—we see the self as originally an extension of experience of the other" (Fonagy *et al.*, 2002). Without this experience, the sense of self is rooted, not in the mind, but in the body. The incapacity to psychologically reflect on and integrate mental experiences results in the person having only the body and bodily experiences through which to provide a sense of relief, release or consolidation. Borderline, perverse and violent patients often speak of a profound sense of relief and peace following an act of violence or a suicide attempt.

The lack of a containing function leaves persecutory and toxic object relationships festering in the mind, constituting a cruel and threatening presence that has to be annihilated for self-preservation. The capacity to deal with this psychologically is non-existent or extremely fragile. It can only be dealt with physically, using the body. If projected, it may result in a sadistic, violent or murderous attack on the body of the victim. If identified with, it becomes masochistic or results in a suicidal attack on the physical self.

In thinking about failure in containment and the resulting sado-masochistic and violent interactions, we should probably also keep in mind the nature of the death instinct, which, at its strongest, attacks and distorts the capacities for perception and judgement, both in the potentially available containing object and in the self. It is a useful construct if it is thought of as a destructive *psychological* force (Segal, 1993; Feldman, 2000). What is deadly about the death instinct is the way in which meaning, and specifically difference, is attacked, resulting in the retardation of the development of a thinking psychological self (Feldman, 2000) and hence creating what Chasseguet-Smirgel calls the perverse patient's "substitute reality" (reported in Leigh, 1998).

Summary

We might say that our Oedipal destiny obliges us to manage, tolerate and find creative expression for our aggressive and loving feelings in relation to the realities of life, especially those of dependence, the double difference between the sexes and the generations and the inevitability of loss. This involves giving up narcissism and omnipotence, recognizing our dependence on others, and tolerating loss, all of which require us to contain the inevitable feelings of ambivalence, of love and hate, separateness, difference and gratitude. If this can be achieved the interlacing of sex and aggression becomes available for expression in the service of creativity and passion in whatever arenas of life and relationships.

If, however, the lack or failure of containment, resulting in an incapacity for mentalization, combined with the strength of the death instinct, does not allow for the toleration of these fundamental facts of life, the aggression aroused recruits sexuality and becomes acted out, defensively, in sado-masochistic, perverse or violent ways. The interlacing of sex and aggression is then recruited in the service of the hostile disavowal of the facts of life, and is destructive of the realities of life and of the creative potential of relationships.

Note

This chapter was previously published in *Aggression and Destructiveness: Psychoanalytic Perspectives*, Celia Harding (Ed.), London and New York: Routledge, 2006. Parts of this chapter were previously published in a paper titled "States of mind in perversion and violence" in *The Journal of the British Association of Psychotherapists*, *41*(2), July 2003.

CHAPTER THREE

The internal couple and the Oedipus complex in cases of perversion

David Morgan

In psychoanalysis a person's first relationships and how they are experienced are seen as the bedrock of future psychic and sexual life. This is a complex interaction between the child and the parental couple, starting with mother. Mother acts as a container for her child's fears, anxieties and desires. Her capacity to bear these powerful impulses relates to her own internal objects and external relationships.

Understanding the complexity of the child's mind and social world began with Freud's theory of the Oedipal complex. In Sophocles' myth, Oedipus encounters the parental couple, unknowingly committing the murder of his father and incest with his mother. He destroys his father, i.e. excludes him, and forms an exclusive link to his mother. The common denominator in all Oedipal configurations involves an attempt to split the parental couple, but with a hope that the parental couple will manage this attack without either excluding the child or colluding. It includes the denial of differences of the generation gap, a wish to create a world where differences are eliminated.

Children's experience of their parents as a couple and the type of relationships they have as adults are linked. Freud emphasised the sexual aspect of the Oedipus complex. Its conflicts, under castration threats, were partially resolved by identification with the same-sex parent, the formation of the superego, and the establishment of the incest taboo towards the parent of the opposite sex. Melanie Klein deepened our understanding of what underpins the Oedipus complex. It is not only the threat of castration that makes the child renounce the parents as sexual objects: the active desire to love and tolerate frustration enables the child to allow the parents their creativity and to become creative himself. In Kleinian thinking the couple becomes an internal object, which develops partly from experiences with the real parents and partly through the complex interaction of love and hate, guilt, reparative feelings, towards not one parent or the other but the link between them. That the child is created by a couple is a powerful truth. At the deepest level, realising that one's life began as an act of love and ecstasy between two people is the optimal start in life.

After conception and birth, the child needs to be contained. In psychoanalysis containment means:

> when an infant has an intolerable anxiety he deals with it by projecting it into the mother. The mother's response is to acknowledge the anxiety and do whatever is necessary to relieve the infant's distress. The infant's perception is that he has projected something intolerable into his object, but the object was capable of containing it and dealing with it. He is then able to re-introject not only his original anxiety, but an anxiety modified by having been contained. He also introjects an object capable of containing and dealing with the anxiety. The containment of anxiety in this way is the beginning of mental stability. This stability can be disrupted due to the mother being unable to bear the prejected anxiety so that the infant introjects an experience of even greater terror than the one he has projected. It may also be disrupted by excessive destructive omnipotence of the infant's fantasy.
>
> [Segal, 1975, pp. 134–135]

This containment includes child and mother, the child and mother's world, including her own mind and needs, father, friends and other helpmates: from the beginning of life there is an interplay that involves at least three people. The child learns that this is manageable or feels excluded and vulnerable, leading to conflict and anxiety.

Within this constellation the child projects into mother an image of its own anxiety. If mother is experienced as an object that cannot manage more than one relationship at a time, the child may feel that only an exclusive relationship is possible. The mother's needs or her involvement with others—other children or partner—can be experienced as intrusive, threatening to exclude the child. This interplay is the beginning of a complex inter-dynamic social relationship. The object is explored intimately to discover in it the capacity to bear conflict, which the child as yet cannot. Recognition of the parental sexual relationship involves relinquishing the idea of sole and permanent possession of mother, leading to a profound sense of loss, which, if not tolerated, may become a sense of persecution. How this is experienced underpins all future mental and emotional life (Britton, 1989).

To cope with this profound sense of loss the child needs to project his own terror of abandonment into his objects. When his projection is met, the child is enabled to work through the feelings of love, hatred and guilt, which he projected into the couple. Then the link between the mother and the father is seen as positive and creative, rather than destructive and excluding.

The mixture of a person's reality and fantasy concerning the parental relationship effects and underpins the quality of all their future relationships, the nature of their anxieties and defences, and profoundly effects their capacity for creative thinking. In fantasy, the parental couple can be experienced as coming together in lively and pleasurable or destructive ways and these will determine the way a person experiences things coming together in his own mind, his own thoughts, or relationships. The capacities to think and to relate to a parental couple are thus connected. Thinking about the other, in this case the parents, is the prototype of all future mental and sexual life: how I think about you thinking about me affects my own thoughts about myself. Klein suggested that this process of thinking about their parents and how they feel responded to, begins in the infant's earliest moments of life. The infant always relates to an object such as the breast, or other parts such as the mother's mind, but there are always other objects, atmospheres and presences representing the other. The infant's experiences of these interactions form the child's attitude and relationship to this unfolding experience, laying the foundation for the urge and capacity to learn, to know, and to relate to reality. Klein later described this as the depressive position—a realization of the real world outside the self, the difference between internal and external. The Oedipus situation is an exploration of the other, beginning with the child's recognition of the parents' relationship in whatever primitive or partial form. This is followed by rivalry with one parent for the other. It is resolved when the child relinquishes his claim on his parents by accepting the reality of their sexual relationship.

Britton (1989) designated three positions for the child within the triangular situation:

1. having a separate link with each of the parents;
2. being the observer of but non-participant in their relationship;
3. being observed by them.

Accepting this link, that couples get together to make babies, is difficult: it excludes and exclusion can only be managed by attacking and destroying any representation of the parental couple, or, as in psychosis, by attacking all links so that nothing gets together to make anything else.

Anxiety becomes the parent's responsibility, to be resolved in the parent's mind or heart before it is returned to the child. To be digestible and helpful, the child has to feel that the parent has been able to ameliorate these powerful feelings in a non-persecutory way. This interaction is the foundation of all future intercourse: if I put part of myself into the other, how it is received involves exploration, tenderness and love, as well as sadism, penetration and hate. The parents' capacity to resolve this dilemma depends on their own Oedipal experiences. If the parent is a member of a mature couple in their own mind, including their own internal couple and relationship to a partner, a child's fantasies need not be denied or acted out. This capacity, or later *in loco parentis*, the analyst's capacity, to think rather than act, communicates that there is help at hand: there is another object in their mind to which they can turn, so they are not overwhelmed, unlike the child.

In analysis this conflict often occurs: a patient angrily retorts in a Friday session about the weekend, "when you leave me, I feel you don't give a damn about me, you are with your family and they are more important to you than me". To reassure the patient would be a lie: the analyst's family, in reality, is more important to him than the patient, particularly at the weekend. The patient would triumph over the analyst's family, forming an idealised transference with a lonely old analyst who had nobody else but her. Confirming the patient's fears that she is meaningless is equally untrue; our patients mean a lot to us, analysis is an intense attachment. The painful triangular reality can be recognised, hopefully in a helpful way, by saying "You feel that because I have people in my life other than you, you no longer feature as an important person in my mind at all." In this way the analyst meets the patient's projections of her rivalry and jealousy by thinking both about her and about the others in his life without excluding her. A link is made rather than destroyed. A patient recently responded to a weekend by dreaming of a couple on a train bound for Russia. He was relieved to discover that the train was in fact bound for Middlesex, a county adjoining his—representing the bedroom next door—making a link between himself and the parental couple.

Over many such interactions, an internal model of mental intercourse can be established, representing the parents' good sexual intercourse, tolerating anxiety, dependency and separateness. When I have an anxiety I can turn for help in my mind to a creative intercourse with my wife, analyst, supervisor and psychoanalytical theory. If this is a creative experience, thoughts and ideas can interact in a kind of healthy intercourse. Conversely, a bizarre or predominately destructive couple, or an analyst who is vulnerable and alone, might have little capacity to turn to another: this can lead to damaged, perverse or inhibited forms of relating and thinking. This constellation is frequently found in inexperienced clinicians who, from kindness or the need to reassure the patient, allow an unanalysed positive transference to develop as if to meet the patient's fantasies of their total devotion. This can lead patients to believe that an overly involved therapist has met their projections, or therapists to identify with the projection by thinking they are indispensable to the patient. Alternatively, the analyst may respond in over-rigid ways encouraging the patient to conform.

A patient group illustrates what happens when the internal couple becomes pathological: patients with various problems show the many permutations or perversions of this early blueprint. In these cases we can discern a continuum from the earliest breakdown in

Oedipal relations—such as fearing engulfment by mother in the absence of father, or an attacking mother personifying her child's projections of his own aggression—to later developments where the relationship to mother is fairly resolved but the connection to father is faulty.

- A trans-sexual man wants to remove his old man (penis) surgically and fulfil his wish to become a woman. He portrays his mother as encouraging him to become a woman, and his father as violent; he wishes to dis-identify with his father and identify with mother by literally getting inside her.
- Further along this continuum is a transvestite man who imagines getting in and out of women's clothes at will. He does not want to stay inside a woman's body forever as it becomes a claustrophobic trap threatening to engulf him. However he uses it to make his wife feel second class and triumphs over her as his accomplice. In his internal couple mother is frightening and powerful, over-involved with her son, sometimes exciting him, sometimes ignoring him. Meanwhile father is inadequate and uninvolved.
- A homosexual man cruises, exposing himself to AIDS by compulsively engaging in unprotected sex. He has a good relationship with mother, but feels his father was dictatorial. A sexually abusive father-figure, a priest, compounds the picture of frightening men. This provides an unreliable internal couple, leading to negation of women and identifications with sexually sadistic men.

These permutations in sexual orientation clearly resonate with an adult's conception of his parents' interactions.

Analysis with patients is a way of exploring the other in an attempt to resolve these conflicts. The analytic mind that encourages lively intercourse must be positively narcissistic, able to meet its own needs, able to relate to others, and, consequently, able to think about the patient. Initially any hint of others in the analyst's life is seen as destructive and excluding, repeating the earliest experience of the breast: the patient often lives in an all or nothing world, feeling that when his object has others, he has no-one. In reality, if the analyst had no-one but his patients, they would be left with an impoverished object unable to help anyone, let alone himself. But the mind projected into the analyst is incapable of thinking of the patient, oneself and the other: it is as if the patient has not experienced a mind with room for all three. This is a projective identification of the patient's own conflict and the analyst is only equipped to respond when his needs—such as family, partner, friends, his own analysis—provide him with experiences of being thought about and an internal world involving intercourse and links with others. This world does not preclude others; indeed a good relationship with another, like the mother with the father, creates the resources for caring for another, rather than becoming over-dependent on the child. This latter might seem desirable to the child but generates confusions between the child's needs and the parent's needs.

Various permutations of the internal couple

Case study one

> A young woman with a needle phobia, starting analysis, dreams that mother sends her to a man for a series of painful injections. It appears from her history that her parents married precipitously after the death of her maternal grandmother when mother was 16 years old. Her parents separated upon the patient's 16th birthday. She dealt with losing the couple by taking the absent father's place and becoming her mother's partner. She thereby denied her father's absence, disposing of her need for a strong father by destroying him and projecting her own needs into her mother. She felt that psychoanalysis was a cruel invasive treatment, that I would use my potency to harm her. This young woman feared intercourse because she feared giving up the potent feelings she derived from looking after mother. She feared becoming a victim of an unscrupulous analyst, who would use her to carry his own pain, whilst making himself feel stronger at her expense, thereby re-enacting what had happened when her parents' marriage ended. The analysis involved undoing this without making her feel I was using my position to hurt and rob her.

Case study two: A transsexual fantasy

> Toni requested a meeting feeling that an assessment might help her confusion over her sexual identity. She told me she was a girl but was confused by wishing to be a boy. When she arrived for her first meeting with me I met a person who could have been either sex. I felt some confusion, in my counter-transference, about whether a boy or girl was peeking out at me from behind this figure. She said she had always been confused about her identity. She had considered a gender reassignment but felt this was too drastic and she knew that it took more to change sex than an operation; in fact it was really rather impossible. She knew it was about something else but didn't know what. She also said that her breasts had not developed and her periods had not started although there were no medical reasons for this.
>
> Her earliest memory was of her father dying when she was two. She told me, proudly, that he was a successful architect and some of his buildings were still standing. Her mother had remarried. Before this Toni felt that she looked after her mother. She did well academically, and won all the races against the boys. She became so good at tennis that she was banned from the all-men's tennis championship because she could have won. She was now a computer expert.
>
> She told me in a rather touching way that, since the age of 4, she had been fascinated by astronomy and begged her mother for a telescope. Since then she had bought three telescopes, each bigger than the one before. Now she had a very large one. She was sure that there was life out there somewhere in the universe and that she would find it someday. She said this with enthusiasm, yet I felt enormously sad and tears came to my eyes. I found myself thinking about my own children whom I hadn't seen all day.

The patient's first communications in psychoanalysis are often the most telling; all are incontrovertible facts and communications about the patient's internal world, connecting us with the patient's unconscious. Toni is telling me about her confusion, ostensibly about her sexual identity, and she tells me the story of her life as she sees it. It involves a mother, and a father who dies before she feels they know each other. Her mother is depressed and Toni feels responsible for her, becoming in some ways her partner and caretaker. One understanding of this would be that her loss of her father, and guilt that her rivalry with him for mother killed him, is projected into her mother who is understandably depressed at this time. Toni avoids her own feelings by adopting the position of mother's partner, the lost father, feeling like a male. Her own need for father is expressed by identifying with him, attempting to keep him alive by taking him into her own body. The telescopes are symbols of potency, as is her sad search for life in space, for the lost father. My own counter-transference reactions to the story suggest that she is unconscious of her sadness over the loss of, and her confusion about, the absent father. I interpreted that I felt she longed for her father to fill the empty space his absence created; that she dealt with this feeling by caring for her mother who also missed him. One way of caring for her mother and herself was to become a male that both of them lost, and keep him alive in that way. She looked thoughtful for a moment and said, "Phew, that's a bit Freudian". She was right: I was thinking about her problem as an unresolved Oedipal situation. She managed her pain and confusion by freeze-framing a part of her mind and body at a time when the conflict over her own sexual identity occurred.

Case study three: An unresolved homosexual anxiety

Mr C. loved his wife very much but he was obsessed by thoughts of golden-haired young men with whom he was driven to perform oral sex. He had these thoughts only when making love to his wife. He found them depressing, felt paranoid about them and wondered if he had an unconscious wish to be gay. Mr C. said he loved his parents. He was the eldest, close to his mother, but longed for a closer relationship with his father. His father, a sporting person, seemed to devote all his energies to his younger son, a "blonde hairdo" surfer type. Even though Mr C. was more successful than his brother he felt that his father never gave him the recognition he deserved. Exploring this in the transference revealed his craving for recognition from his father and me. He dealt with his rivalry with his brother for father by projecting the unwanted feelings into the woman, giving all his desire at moments of intimacy to the golden boy image that his father had idealised. Exploring this with me helped him feel that I was not seduced by this idealised image that he felt he had to suck up to, and that I could appreciate a real him. Consequently he felt more attentive with his wife and after a while his ambivalence towards her disappeared, as did his homosexual longings. He felt his father did not

> provide an alternative to his mother's love. Feeling rejected by father, he turned against his wife (and probably his mother) joining his father's latent narcissistic longings expressed through his golden boy son. Discovering that his rivalous and desirous feelings towards his father's favourite boy underpinned his longings for the gay encounter enabled him to feel sad about his father's apparent immaturity but enabled him to love and appreciate his wife again. He later talked to his father who told him that he had always felt inferior to his own brother, whom his father had loved more than him. He was mortified to learn that he had maybe recreated this with his son.

I will end this paper with a detailed analysis of a patient with a perverse fantasy in which the analysis of the internal couple played a significant role. I will highlight the use of the transference in bringing these conflicts to the fore, and how the analyst's mind recreates the patient's earliest conflicts, leading to some reparation of the couple in the patient's mind and consequently an improvement in his capacity to relate socially and sexually.

Case study four: Psychoanalysis of a transvestite fantasy

> Mr D is 30 years old and started analysis five years ago. He came into treatment feeling confused and depressed because his wife refused to continue to participate in his transvestite activity and was threatening to leave. He felt she was unreasonable and was attacking him. In addition, he wanted to be a writer but he only wrote articles for women's magazines, which were always rejected. He lived on a trust fund left to him by his mother's father, in a house that was purchased for him. He paid for his analysis from this fund. He was aware of feeling depressed and lethargic, as if all the energy was in everyone else. I gleaned that Mr D had felt lonely in his early childhood. He remembered having a rubber sheet that comforted him as a baby and child. I feel that this could be seen as his defensive retreat, to a reliable object that he could control and comfort himself. This attachment to materials intensified later into a secret wish to dress up in his mother's clothes. He described a sense of calm that would descend on him at these times.
>
> Mr D is the eldest of three children. His father was an accountant who abandoned the family when he was implicated for fraud. Mr D., who was three at the time, did not see his father again until, as a result of his analysis, he decided to find and confront him. Mother

appears to have become depressed and unavailable when the marriage ended. Mr D felt it was his responsibility to put away childish things, and set an example to his siblings by caring for his mother. He can remember how responsible he felt on the one hand, and on the other hand, feeling numb and desperately trying to hold on to reality. He found the experience of putting on and taking off his mother's clothes extremely gratifying, relieving him from confusion.

His mother remarried when he was fourteen, to a man he respects but whom he experienced as a disciplinarian. When he changed his name to his step-father's he felt further distanced from his own identity. His step-father encouraged him to study at school and this helped him get to university. However, he soon found the work dense and difficult and barely got his degree. He felt increasingly lethargic when he started a postgraduate degree in philosophy. He found Western philosophy impenetrable and retreated into Indian mysticism. He tended to attract younger students, becoming something of a guru in the students' union. He dropped out of this course eventually suffering from migraines and unable to think.

He married a student from abroad who became very dependent on him. She was abused sexually by her father when she was five. Within this relationship they regressed to an internal world inside his house, living on his trust fund. He drew her into his transvestite activities, dressing up as a woman and masturbating in front of her. He felt this gave him power over her that comforted him. Here we see him prejecting his needy infantile self into her whilst he becomes the provider. His wife's subsequent refusal to participate in this arrangement distressed him. His fragile world was collapsing. He described feeling almost catatonic with depression, raising himself from this torpor only to eat or evacuate.

He spent a great deal of time at home trying to write articles for women's magazines: a concrete form perhaps of getting parts of his mind into women. However, they were always rejected. In frustration he berated his wife, often violently, for being stupid and lazy. He was able to do this partly as she was still a student, as stuck as he was. He kept her financially and threatened her with eviction. Since they married their sexual relationship was minimal except for the transvestite activity. She seemed at first willing to play the voyeur to his exhibitionism, presumably re-enacting her own abuse by her father.

Here we can see Mr D projecting his infantile self into his wife. She has to stay in this position lest she threaten him with awareness of his own needs, whilst he retains the power to look after her or abandon her. Thus, his own experiences are reversed and projected into his wife, who was always frightened that he would leave. As we can see, the damaged or absent maternal object is replaced almost entirely in fantasy by the subject so that whilst he feels in control, other people like his wife are reduced to the role of an accomplice. He reverses earlier experiences of deprivation through putting them physically and psychologically into the body and mind of the other. He aims to evacuate his unwanted parts so forcefully into the other that the communicative aspect of the projections is unlikely to be recognised. His wife's experience of abuse made her an available recipient of his projections.

In the first year of analysis Mr D was increasingly fearful about his needy self surfacing. He became enormously anxious about becoming addicted to his analysis, which he said was an arrangement that would rob him of his autonomy. He felt that I was intent on seducing him into a relationship with me so that I could use him entirely for my own ends without considering him. He was convinced of the accuracy of his perceptions and oblivious to the irony that they contained a mirror image of how he used his wife. I interpreted these anxieties saying that he feared a rather empty analyst whose own life was so devoid of any real substance that I derived my only comfort by seducing and controlling my patients into providing me with the feelings of power lacking in my impoverished life. He was interested in these observations and curious at my willingness to be explored as such an unattractive figure. He became less anxious and more able to explore what realities these accusations might have.

Analysing the internal couple around the breaks was crucial in managing his acting out. As he became more aware of his dependence on me, his fury with his wife increased. After a Bank Holiday weekend he felt enraged with her saying she was a bloodsucker. It was as if she was a parasite that he felt like killing to protect himself. He comforted himself through dressing up and masturbating. Thus, he simultaneously projected his own emerging dependency into his wife whilst he, in fantasy, became the mother. He then felt ambivalent about returning to his analysis, wanting to stay in bed rather than attend sessions. I showed him how, at these times, I am the abandoning father leaving him alone with his wife/mother into whom he projects his own needs. He can avoid needing me, both by gratifying himself and by evacuating all his neediness into his wife. He fears my return because the analysis will put him in touch with his own needy self and a vengeful me who feels robbed by a "him" who has taken over my qualities and put his wife in the patient's position. I also connected this ambivalence and fear to his mother's second husband who pushed him out of the nest.

As I encouraged him to think about, rather than enact, these things he became very critical of his analyst. He attempted to take his feelings outside the analysis and dump them into his wife. However, he felt less convinced by what he was doing to her and she seemed more able to resist it. He furiously attacked me, certain of my perverse aims: "Wasn't Freud a charlatan anyway?" He voraciously devoured negative reports in the papers and quoted the writings of critics of psychoanalysis at me. He was also at these times fond of calling me "a complete cunt". I was eventually able to take up his anxiety that I was unreal. I was a man dressed up in the clothing of psychoanalysis, a discredited theory used as a way to control him. He responded by attacking his wife again. She was infuriating, driving him mad with "his" incessant demands. He was unaware of this slip. I said that although he located this needy baby-self in his wife, he was also aware that these feelings belonged to him: he feared his need for me would drive me away (like his father), so he put them into his wife where he could control them. I thought he was searching for a mind that could contain and understand his evacuated feelings of abandonment and loss rather than become identified with them, like his mother and wife, or reject him by walking out, like his father.

After the third year there was an important development. His need to project the unwanted aspects of himself into his wife, who was becoming stronger, abated. He became terrified that he was going to slip into a massive depression. He dreamt of falling, of losing his grip, of being lost at sea with a lighthouse in the distance, of losing himself in the underground. These dreams suggest original fears of disintegration, of the overwhelming mother and the distant unavailable father who might have been able to throw light on his predicament and save him. His fears of being engulfed by a void felt palpable and we were confronted by the possibility that he might break down. Mindful of the attacks that he might make on his wife, I feared she could become the recipient of his breaking down self. He had a powerful wish to impregnate his wife, despite her wishes, thinking this would provide relief from his own feelings. I showed him that he wished to get rid of his childlike feelings in his analysis by puffing them physically into his wife, impregnating her with his split-off self, enacting the transvestite's wish to occupy mother. Thus his wish to evacuate this part of himself into the mother/wife was contained in the transference with me, rather than being enacted, leading to a possible conception. (How many children are created for this reason?)

At this time he had a dream confirming his emerging baby-like feelings and his wish to be rid of them. He is living in a flat on the set of Eldorado, the soap opera that flopped. He is with his wife. He thinks it is wonderful but a child looks into the window of the flat and he feels terrified that it will get in and take over. The flat is taken over by lots of children and he and his wife are overwhelmed. I said that his dependency with me frightened him because he feared that I might not be able to cope.

A week later he reported a second dream. He is again in a flat in Eldorado with his wife but this time he is aware of being frightened. The whole set is on fire. He realises this is just a superficial film set and, as it is about to collapse, the Prince of Wales rescues him. As soon as they are out of danger, the Prince (a reference to my Welshness or baldness) is occupied by two children. I said that although Mr D felt rescued by me from the dangerous illusion that he lives in with his wife and mother, I quickly abandon him, like father, for people I deem to be more interesting than him. He knows that he needs his father's help to leave the fantasy world where he has been living with his mother but, like his father, I will leave him for other children. Around this time he discovered where his father lived and, amidst great pain and sadness, found he was remarried with two children.

As a result of meeting his father and the gradual strengthening of his wife and me in his mind, his terror of his neediness returned. He dreamt that his wife was a vampire. She bites him and he becomes a vampire too. I feel this vampire is a perverse image of the sucking baby. The source of evil is now in them both. They search a jungle for the source of evil to save themselves. They see a huge stone statue of Orson Welles, the outside shell crumbles and it comes alive. They become aware that this is the source of all evil. In the dream he attacks it and cuts it to pieces. I feel this dream illustrates Mr D's dilemma. He needs an object into whom he can project the cannibalistic parts of himself but he fears they will then hunt and kill him. I said to him that when I leave him, he becomes frightened and confused by his relationship with his wife, as he did with his mother when they both felt like needy children. He is aware of how much they need a third person to help them. However, rather than a helpful person who can think about this with him, I become full of the cruelty that he fears so much, so he can justifiably destroy me.

At this time he decided to get a job. He now only used the cross-dressing in the analytic breaks. He seemed to be aware that I might be able to think about his needs rather than be overwhelmed or rejecting of him. He had reached the point where he could explore the realities of his projections in his analyst, rather than put them into an object that could not help him understand, like his wife or mother.

During a weekend break, having berated his wife again he had a dream. He is on a working holiday in the USA, in the desert, and is worried that he is short of money. It becomes rather like a "Mad Max" movie. His mother appears, as if by magic, with a credit store card for Selfridges. After initial relief he is shocked to find a credit limit of fifty pounds. I said that he deals with the painful reality of losing his father and me by rewriting a mad story of himself and his mother, living in a state of perpetual bliss, which he can use like his cross-dressing, to avoid doing any real work. However, he is aware that this makes a limiting desert of his life. He responded by saying that he had told his wife that he had made a will that no one could benefit from, including her. He had been surprised when she cried. I said that rather than understand this problem in himself, he makes out that other people are interested in free-loading on him. He believes that he is taking care of others as a way of avoiding getting on with his own life, recreating his time with mother when she might have depended on him. His wife then has to tolerate having his dependency needs being pushed into her whilst he has none at all.

Now that Mr D can hear my communications, he is more aware of his own destructiveness. In a Friday session he presented material that was about painful separation and the role of the internal couple in his internal world. He dreamt that he was going away with me but that I give him a false address. He runs to the station but sees me leaving with my wife and realises he is being left behind. I said that it was painful when, like the false father, I leave him. He feels that if things were different I would take him with me. I felt he was more aware of the importance of his analysis and beginning to be aware of an Oedipal couple. On Monday he reported a terrifying nightmare about death: "My mother is dying of cancer. I have a child and I am trying to take care of it. My fear is that he is dying too. I take some of my mother's medicine and give it to the child." I said that during the break he was so furious with me for leaving him that he kills off his analysis. He then discovers that not only is his analysis dying but also the life that he has started here with me. His fears of dying surfaced and his feelings of dependency, on his wife and analyst, intensified.

In a final weekend dream he demonstrates his psychotic anxieties

> and his dependency on me. He dreams he is sitting on top of a monument that changes suddenly into a collapsing black industrial chimney. Someone passes him a rope and he climbs out. I said that on the weekend he climbs on top of his analysis but becomes frightened of being stuck inside something dead and collapsing about him, the dead body of the triumphed-over mother. He is relieved by the return of his analysis on Monday because it and I are still alive.

I believe this dream reflects a change in his view of the internal couple: instead of being left inside the dead body of a mother he is rescued by a father with a penis. Now he is more aware of what he does to his objects, taking over their good qualities and evacuating what is felt to be bad into them. I think he is genuinely relieved and hopeful that someone can save him from this.

The analysis has helped Mr D to feel that I can bear becoming what he projects into me long enough to explore and contain these elements. His has less need to evacuate into an object that is unable to understand him and is able to project into someone who is better able to understand his communications and return them to him in a digestible form. An important part of this work is the capacity of the analyst to bear the projections long enough for the patient to discover whether the analyst corresponds to them or not. They can then be interpreted to the patient, who can begin to symbolise them (rather than enact them) through other forms of communication such as dreams. The inevitable attack and destruction of the other can then be avoided and something more creative can be, hopefully, allowed to develop.

Note

This chapter was previously published in *Sexuality: Psychoanalytic Perspectives*, Celia Harding (Ed.), London and New York: Routledge, 2001.

CHAPTER FOUR

Psychoanalytic contributions to risk assessment and management

Jessica Yakeley

Introduction

Dangerousness and madness have long been linked in the collective imagination, inspiring film and literature, fuelling the media and providing both fascination and fear for the general public. Although there is only a slightly increased, albeit significant, risk of violence amongst people with more serious mental disorders (Taylor and Estroff, 2003), in recent years, considerations of risk have become of central importance to all those working in the field of mental health. The closure of the old mental asylums and release of patients into a community that was insufficiently equipped to contain them, resulted in some highly publicized failures of community care in which serious incidents occurred (Reed, 1997). The ensuing public inquiries condemning the inadequate assessment of patients and the poor communication amongst the mental health professionals and other agencies involved, have created a culture of blame in which politicians and public alike appear more concerned with public protection than with the individual rights of the mentally ill patient. The waters become even muddier when the offender's mental state and behaviour do not fit neatly into a psychiatric diagnostic category but are attributed to an abnormality of character. Public outrage over sex-offenders and so-called "dangerous severe personality disorder" have contributed to the recent proposals for legislation requiring psychiatrists to forcibly detain people who may commit some dangerous act in the future but have not done so yet. Understandable though these anxieties might be, they have the capacity to seriously damage progress towards less authoritarian and custodial mental health services. This is of relevance not only in the forensic mental health services but in all mental health and psychotherapeutic practice.

In this chapter I would like to consider the assessment of dangerousness from a psychoanalytic perspective. Psychoanalysts and psychoanalytic psychotherapists may not be routinely involved in day to day decision making involving risk in mental health services, and it might be assumed that patients in psychotherapeutic treatment pose minimal risk. The psychotherapist, however, is no longer confined to her ivory tower. The last decade has witnessed the advent of a new sub-specialty within psychiatry, forensic psychotherapy, and in non-forensic psychiatric settings psychotherapists are being increasingly referred patients with complex psychopathology and acting-out behaviours. The psychodynamic psychotherapist can contribute to thinking about dangerousness at different levels and across different mental health settings, not only through the direct assessment and treatment of patients, but also by supervising, teaching and consulting to other mental health workers.

I am not advocating that a psychoanalytic approach should replace conventional risk assessment but I want to highlight how certain psychoanalytic concepts can enhance thinking about risk. Fundamental to this approach is the attempt to understand and find meaning in the anti-social act, specifically the unconscious meaning that is not available to the violent person—that which is unbearable to think finds its expression in action.

Models of risk

The current preoccupation with the prediction of violence in the users of services for the mentally ill has led to the development of formal tools for the assessment of risk in such populations. There are two main models of risk assessment—the mathematical or actuarial, and the clinical (Buchanan, 1999). Clinicians have traditionally assessed risk on the basis of individual clinical judgement. The unstructured clinical approach, however, has been criticized for its low validity, low inter-rater reliability and poor predictive value. The realization that the prediction of dangerousness is notoriously unreliable (Monahan, 1984) has led to the introduction of structured risk assessment forms into many mental health services, such as the Care Programme Approach (CPA), and these encourage staff to think about risk and to collect historical data.

More recent research prioritizes an actuarial model of risk assessment over clinical judgement. The actuarial assessment of risk originated in the insurance industry and is an epidemiologically-based approach which studies relevant populations to develop structured risk assessment schedules which are standardized to the particular population, for example, prison inmates, or patients in a medium secure unit. The actuarial tool collects mainly static data about the patient, such as demographic variables, which are known to predict violence across settings and individuals, and can be coded in a predetermined manner and a formula applied to give a predictive value for a future act of violence. Such static variables known to increase the risk of future violence would include previous episodes of violence, being male, being of lower intelligence, low socio-economic status and drug or alcohol abuse. The actuarial approach, however, cannot identify the triggers to the violent act in any particular individual, nor can it examine how a violent person's history, environment and current relationships, including professional care, interact to influence his behaviour. Thus the actuarial method, whilst improving consistency of risk prediction across groups, tends to ignore individual variations in risk by failing to prioritize clinically relevant variables and minimizing the role of clinical judgement.

Clinical example

Ms L, a young woman from a middle-class family, had a history of self-harm, but no violence towards others, and was receiving psychotherapy. During a break in therapy due to the therapist's planned vacation she killed a member of her extended family. Had she been

> assessed with an actuarial scale prior to the killing she would have scored as being of very low risk, as she was female, middle class, and had no history of violence to others. However, in retrospect it was possible to understand this murderous act in the context of unconscious feelings of abandonment and rage related to early parental abuse that were reactivated in the transference due to the therapist's absence and enacted in her violence with fatal consequences.

Researchers in the field of psychiatric risk assessment have recognized some of the limitations of the actuarial method and have incorporated more dynamic clinical variables into risk prediction instruments. Risk scales have proliferated and been implemented in almost all mental health services in recent years, creating a mountain of paperwork for clinicians to complete, some would argue at the expense of talking to patients. Moreover, these risk assessment schedules do not include any attempt to consider the unconscious variables that may crucially influence the violent act. Such unconscious motivations can only be assessed by clinical contact with individual patients and attempting to enter into the internal world of the offender, a task that may understandably be resisted by many who fear the physical and emotional risks that such a clinical encounter entails. Indeed, the predictive approach can be seen as a defence against coming into real contact with violent patients (Doctor, 2003). Instead it is proposed that the role of clinical experience should regain its centrality in the assessment and management of dangerousness. This experience is the unique encounter between two individuals in which the unconscious meaning of violent acts and feelings can be explored between patient and therapist within the arenas of transference and counter-transference in a safe therapeutic setting. One of the truisms in risk assessment is that the best predictor of future behaviour is previous behaviour. But this historical pattern can only form a context in which the present and future can be understood. Prediction of the triggers and timing of a violent act can be enhanced by an understanding of the complexity of conscious and unconscious communications of the violent patient, and how his reactions to the environment are influenced by unconscious processes that are determined by his history.

Definitions of risk

The term risk is increasingly used in clinical practice in preference to the more subjective and pejorative label of dangerousness. This change in terminology in itself creates the illusion that risk is a statistical fact based on objective assessment. But what is the risk being considered? What is its nature, severity or frequency? Risk is often defined in terms of an event outcome, such as violence towards others or towards oneself, but prior to this there are numerous risk-influencing factors that need consideration, such as non-compliance with medication, relapse of a mental illness or disengagement from therapy. Such factors contribute to the overall process of risk assessment as the patient moves through the pathway of care (Antebi, 2003). Many of these factors cannot be measured by risk assessment schedules, but can only be assessed and evaluated through understanding the patient's history and current functioning in the context of the therapeutic relationship.

Considerations of risk have traditionally been subdivided into risk assessment, risk management and risk prevention. But clinical experience shows that the assessment of risk is an ongoing process that forms an integral part of the risk management and containment of the patient. Treatment which is aimed at reducing risk in the long term may actually increase risk in the short term as the patient becomes aware of previously repressed painful thoughts and feelings which cannot be tolerated and are enacted in violence. This does not only occur in those patients receiving psychotherapy, as a necessary process to be worked through, but may be an unexpected adverse result of otherwise seemingly effective medication.

Clinical example

Mr P, a 65-year-old man with a long-standing schizophrenic illness (but no history of self-harm) and Diogenes Syndrome (pathological hoarding), was admitted to a psychiatric hospital under the Mental Health Act after the housing department became concerned that his flat filled with old papers and furniture had become a health and safety hazard. The onset of Mr P's illness appeared to have started after the death of his wife 20 years ago. Mr P presented as a cheerful man, although angry that he had been forcibly removed from his flat where he believed that his wife—the Queen of England—lived with him, the King. His flat was adorned with pictures of the (real) Royal Family. Mr P was treated with anti-psychotic medication and his delusions rapidly evaporated. However, he became increasingly withdrawn and hanged himself a few months later. His psychosis could be seen as protecting him from the painful reality of his wife's death, and once the delusions improved with medication he was overwhelmed with feelings of desperation and anger that were expressed in his suicidal violence.

Violence and acting out

Fundamental to any assessment of how dangerous a person is is an attempt to understand the meaning of their violence. Violence can be understood as a form of "acting out". In his paper "Remembering, repeating and working through" (1914) Freud says,

> The patient does not *remember* anything of what he has forgotten and repressed, but *acts* it out. He reproduces it not as a memory, but as an action: he *repeats* it, without, of course, knowing that he is repeating it. For instance, the patient does not say that he remembers that he used to be defiant and critical towards his parents' authority; instead, he behaves that way to the doctor.

Freud went on to show how acting out was related both to the transference and resistance. The transference could be regarded as a repetition of the patient's past and could result in acting out involving the person of the analyst. "The greater the resistance, the more extensively will acting out (repetition) replace remembering . . . if, as the analysis proceeds, the transference becomes hostile or unduly intense and therefore in need of repression, remembering at once gives way to acting out."

Freud regarded acting out as a clinical psychoanalytic concept related specifically to psychoanalytic treatment. However, the concept has since been widened to include a whole range of impulsive, anti-social and dangerous actions of patients, arising not just as a consequence to the clinical context, but describing habitual modes of action and behaviour resulting from the personality and pathology of the individual. Fenichel (1945) linked impulsive tendencies to difficulties in the first year of life, suggesting that traumatic experiences in childhood may lead to repeated attempts to master, through activity, what was once passively and traumatically experienced. In other words, dangerousness represents an infantile danger that the adult cannot remember but is enacted on an external object as a way of reversing the experience.

The violent act can therefore be viewed as a behaviour that has replaced thinking. Many violent individuals describe how during the actual act of violence they have no thoughts, and often feel frighteningly out of control. One of the tasks of the psychotherapist is to enable the patient to think about the meaning of their violence, to explore the mind of the patient, its unconscious processes and defence mechanisms, and how his or her dangerous behaviour resides in that mind (Minne, 2003).

But this awareness of mind can in itself be perceived as dangerous by patients who may habitually use defensive manoeuvres such as denial, minimization or amnesia to protect them from anxieties about knowing about their actions that they fear could overwhelm them and lead to madness or suicide. Winnicott (1959–1964) described the adult patient's fear of breakdown as representing an original breakdown and failure of defences in infancy, following which new defences were organized constituting the patient's illness pattern or abnormal personality. He regarded adult psychopathy as uncured delinquency that he believed was the result of early childhood deprivation and environmental failure, most importantly inadequate maternal care. Hale (2004) describes the breakdown or dangerous behaviour as occurring when the external reality mirrors the internal feared fantasy.

Self-preservative vs sado-masochistic violence

Glasser's (1998) distinction between two different types of violence, "self-preservative violence" and "sado-masochistic violence", can be helpful in assessing the dangerousness of an individual. He defined violence as an actual assault on the body of one person by another, involving penetration of the body barrier. Self-preservative violence is a primitive response triggered by any threat to the physical or psychological self. Such threats might be external and include the danger of castration, attacks on a person's self-esteem, frustration, humiliation or an insult to an ideal to which the person is attached. The person can also feel threatened by internal sources such as feeling attacked by a sadistic superego or fear a loss of identity by feelings of disintegration and internal confusion. The violent response is fundamental, immediate and aimed at eliminating the source of danger, which may be an external object or an attack on the person's own body which is experienced as a external persecutor in self-harm or suicide.

Sado-masochistic violence is derived from self-preservative violence in that it is a result of the sexualization (a bodily process) of self-preservative violence. This corresponds to the understanding of sadism as the libidinization (a psychic process) of aggression. Sado-masochistic violence is most commonly observed in the perversions, that is people who exhibit a preferred and persistent deviant sexual behaviour that is pervasive and reflects a global structure involving the individual's whole personality. The difference between these two forms of violence is most readily understood by considering their relationship to the object. In self-preservative violence, the object at the time of violence is perceived as being of immediate danger but holds no other personal significance and its responses are of no interest. In sado-masochistic violence, by contrast, the responses of the object are crucial—the object must be seen to suffer, but to do so it must be preserved, rather than eliminated as in the case of self-preservative violence. Sado-masochistic violence also involves pleasure, which is not a component of self-preservative violence. Sado-masochistic violence therefore requires a relationship with another person that involves psychic sado-masochism. A simple example of the difference between the two types of violence would be the soldier who kills the enemy in a battle, believing that such an action is necessary to prevent himself from being killed (self-preservative violence) in contrast to the soldier who captures the enemy and tortures him to make him suffer (sado-masochistic violence).

Self-preservative violence, the aim of which is to eliminate the source of the danger, can therefore be considered more dangerous than sado-masochistic violence, which requires that object to remain alive in order to be controlled and suffer. The same individual can exhibit both forms of violence, which may be thought of as being on a continuum. Sado-masochistic violence can be understood as the more sophisticated reaction, but when it fails it can regress to self-preservative violence. This is very important in considering the risk posed in people with perversions, whose perverse sexual behaviour results from the sexualization of aggression into sadism. Sexualization acts as a binding force in the internal world that enables defensive measures to be more effective and provides a greater sense of stability. It is only when this process breaks down that sadism can revert to aggression, sexual crimes can shade into crimes of violence and the appreciation of the other person as a separate and real object becomes lost.

Clinical example

A psychiatric report was requested to assess risk and inform sentencing for a man on remand charged with sexual assault. He described himself as a professional burglar, but also admitted with some shame and confusion, that he was fascinated by women's underwear. On questioning, he admitted to a sense of sexual excitement on breaking into properties, and on several occasions had felt compelled to rifle through bedroom drawers and had stolen female underwear. On the occasion of the index offence he had broken into and entered a house with the intention of stealing the contents but had been surprised by the owner, an elderly woman. In a panic he tied her up and laid her on the bed where he forced her to take some tablets, thinking they were sleeping pills, so that she would go to sleep. He then felt much calmer and made her strip to her underwear and started masturbating over her panties. When he discovered that she was still awake, he again panicked and tried to hit her; she screamed and struggled, and he ran away feeling terrified. Without speculating about the genesis of his perversion, here it can be seen how in order to control his anxiety and violence he sexualises the situation by attempting to sedate and control the woman by making her unconscious and masturbates over her underwear (sado-masochistic violence) but when she does not comply, he panics, the violence breaks down into self-preservative violence where the source of the danger (the woman with a conscious mind) must be eliminated.

Affect and anxiety in dangerousness

It is important to consider the role of affect and primitive anxieties in the genesis of aggression, an elucidation of which can be crucial in understanding and predicting the triggers to the violent act. Glasser (1979a, 1996) described a particular constellation of interrelated feelings, ideas and attitudes that he called the "core complex", which are fundamental to the pervert's psychopathology. A major component of the core complex is a deep-seated and pervasive longing for an intense and intimate closeness to another person, a wish to merge with them, a "state of oneness" or a "blissful union". Such longings, of course, can occur in all of us, but in the pervert they persist pervasively in a primitive form unmodified by later stages of development. For him, such a merging does not have the quality of a temporary state but is feared as a permanent loss of self, a disappearance of his existence as a separate, independent individual into the object. This anxiety, therefore, is of total annihilation.

To defend against this annihilatory anxiety, the person retreats from the object to a "safe distance". But this flight brings with it feelings of emotional isolation, abandonment, and low self-esteem. These painful feelings prompt the desire for contact and union with the object once more, so that the core complex has the qualities of a vicious circle. The core complex forms a part of normal infantile development where the "object" refers to the mother, but in the pervert, this primitive level of functioning persists and he attempts to resolve his aggression in a very particular way, by sexualization.

Aggression is a central component of the core complex. The annihilatory fear of a loss of separate existence provokes an intense aggressive reaction on the part of the ego. In order to preserve the self, the object—meaning the mother at this very early developmental stage—has to be destroyed. But this of course would mean the loss of all the goodness of the mother, the security, love and warmth that she offers. The pervert attempts to resolve the vicious circle of the core complex by the sexualization of aggression, the conversion of aggression into sadism. The mother is therefore preserved and no longer threatened by total destruction, as the intention to destroy is converted into a wish to hurt and control.

Hale (2004) emphasizes the centrality of affect in the violent act, of which the motivating force is anxiety. He considers each form of dangerousness as having its own different and specific forms of anxiety. Hale divides dangerousness into two types—the perverse, and the violent. In Hale's clinical experience, the perverse dangerous act is triggered by separation anxiety, whereas the fundamental anxiety that triggers an overtly violent response is intrusion (paranoid) anxiety.

These two anxieties, that of abandonment, and that of being engulfed, intruded upon or annihilated, are, of course, the conflicting anxieties that constitute the defensive reactions and vicious circle of the core complex.

Clinical example—perverse dangerousness

A 48-year-old man, Mr D, was referred for psychoanalytic group therapy due to his compulsive use of internet pornography and visits to prostitutes that he felt he had no control over. He was a regular attendee of the group and after several months of therapy proudly announced to the other members of the group that he was no longer resorting to these perverse activities, which he felt had so dominated his life. However, he did not return to the group following a three-week break due to the therapist's annual leave, and the other group members were concerned and wrote to him. After receiving their letter he returned to the group and admitted that he had felt suicidal, taken an overdose and been admitted to a psychiatric ward. He had not made a suicidal attempt since his teenage years when he had felt depressed and abandoned by his mother leaving his father and her children for another man. The group helped Mr D acknowledge that the therapist's leave and the group not meeting had triggered similar feelings of rejection and loss resulting in his suicide attempt, and how his use of pornography and prostitutes had served to protect him from awareness of such painful feelings, as well as providing an outlet for his anger towards his mother that was expressed in his contemptuous attitude towards women.

Clinical example—violent dangerousness

Ms K, a woman in her 40s, was in individual psychodynamic psychotherapy. She had a mother whom she experienced as intrusive and controlling, who then abandoned the family when she was twelve. In her teens and twenties Ms K became violent towards teachers and probation officers, and on one occasion broke into the offices of the probation service to steal her probation records. In therapy, Ms K admitted that she felt violent towards the probation officers as she experienced them as "mind-fuckers" and taking her notes was understood as her attempt to get back her mind from those she perceived as having stolen it from her. This intrusion anxiety, of others entering and controlling her mind as she experienced her mother, was enacted in the transference in her insisting on being accompanied in the sessions by her Alsatian dog. The dog functioned as protecting her from feeling violently intruded upon by the therapist's interpretations as well as protecting the therapist from her own violence.

Gilligan (2000) emphasizes the role that the perception of lack of respect or "disrespect" plays in provoking violence. In working with prison inmates, he was struck by how often these violent men explained their violent assaults by saying they had felt "disrespected", humiliated or shamed. He believes that the emotion of shame is the primary or ultimate cause of all violence, whether towards others or towards the self. Cultural variations in the concepts of shame and honour, for example in Muslim patients, may be important to consider when assessing the triggers to their violence.

When considering risk assessment and psychotherapeutic treatment, it is therefore very important to understand such underlying feelings and anxieties in the patient, and be alert to their appearance in the transference. Professionals are often unaware how breaks in the treatment, for example due to holidays or the clinician leaving the job (for example amongst junior doctors or social workers on short placements in their training), may trigger intense feelings of loss and rejection in the patient who has unconsciously become very dependent on the therapist, key worker, or even institution.

Clinical example

Ms S, a 35-year-old woman with a diagnosis of a borderline personality disorder and history of severe self-harm and violence towards others, had been in conditions of high and then medium security for many years following an offence of arson. Since her admission to an all-female ward in which she received much psychotherapeutic support her mental state and behaviour had improved and she was being considered for discharge into the community, which the patient herself said she desperately wanted. However, in the weeks before her Mental Health Tribunal, Ms S's behaviour deteriorated, she started to cut herself again and staff felt intimidated by her. This pattern of behaviour had been observed in the past when previous discussions regarding discharge had taken place. Here, it can be seen that although Ms S's conscious wish is to live independently in the community, unconsciously she is terrified of this, having become very dependent on the institutional care she has received for so many years. Her dangerous behaviour may be a way of communicating to the staff her (unconscious) anxieties and her wish to remain in a protected environment in which these anxieties can be contained.

Counter-transference

The feelings evoked by the patient in others may provide useful information about the patient's own feelings and state of mind and add a valuable psychoanalytic perspective to the risk assessment of the patient. Counter-transference refers to the thoughts and feelings that the therapist or clinician has towards the patient. Whilst these may reflect the individual therapist's own conflicts and personal history, they may also be a reflection of what the patient feels about, or is doing to, the therapist consciously or unconsciously. The therapist's body and mind can become finely attuned to the mind of the patient such that the unconscious communications of the patient are reflected in the therapist's somatic and affective responses. Awareness of the therapist's counter-transference has become an essential part of the process and technique of modern psychoanalytic therapy and can be used to inform the therapist's therapeutic interventions and interpretations.

Many of the patients we assess find it difficult to tolerate negative feelings such as anger or aggression and the anxiety these provoke, and they can only discharge this anxiety into action, or project it into those around them. These patients, often diagnosed as having borderline, narcissistic or antisocial personality disorders, have poorly developed egos and defences inadequate to contain their impulses, and make excessive use of primitive defence mechanisms such as projection or splitting. Such a patient may claim to be completely unaware of feelings of anxiety or anger, whilst the individuals they come into contact with not only experience these feelings, but are unconsciously nudged into acting them out. This is often explained by the patient's use of the primitive defence mechanism projective identification, first described by Klein (1946), in which the patient externalizes their internal object relationships, which they cannot bear to recognize as internal to themselves and therefore attribute them to others. The person who has been invested with these unwanted aspects may unconsciously identify with what has been projected into them and may be pressurized by the patient to act out in some way. Sandler's (1976) concept of role responsiveness is helpful in further understanding this process. He describes how the patient attempts to bring into reality the self–object interaction represented in the patient's dominant unconscious wishful fantasy. This interaction, involving a role for the subject and another for the object (the role relationship), will tend to be actualized by manipulation of the therapist in the transference via rapid unconscious verbal and non-verbal signals. This pressure from the patient may provoke a particular response in the therapist, leading to counter-transference experiences or even counter-transference enactment by the therapist.

Clinical example

A risk assessment was required on a 78-year-old man, Mr M, who had been admitted to a psychiatric ward following a violent assault on his wife whom he attempted to hit over the head with a hammer when she was asleep. He claimed no recollection of the event. He had a history of heavy alcohol use and bipolar affective disorder, but it appeared that the offence was committed when he was sober and there was no indication that he was suffering a relapse of his mental illness. Tests showed no evidence of organic abnormality or cognitive impairment. Mr M denied any animosity towards his wife and described their marriage in very positive terms, claiming that they never argued. Mrs M initially agreed with her husband when questioned but admitted that in the last year Mr M had become incontinent due to "prostate troubles" and she had become more active in looking after him. Observation of the couple together revealed that she appeared bossy and critical towards her husband and seemed to be the more dominant partner in the relationship, whilst Mr M had a meek and submissive manner tending to agree with everything his wife said. Nursing staff on the ward reported that he was a model patient and considered him a "sweet old man" of low risk, dismissing his offence as an accident that must have occurred when he was half-asleep.

The assessing psychiatrist, however, found herself feeling increasingly impatient with Mr M's repeated refusal to acknowledge any negative feelings towards his wife during their 40-year marriage, despite his mental illness and alcohol abuse. She found herself wanting to "hammer these feelings out of him" and had to make an effort not to appear aggressive or rude in her interactions with the patient. Here we can see that her counter-transference experience represented one side of the unconscious self-object role relationship that Mr M unconsciously sets up, in which a sado-masochistic relation is established between him and his objects. In his interaction with the psychiatrist Mr M denies his own anger and aggression, which are projected into the psychiatrist who then has to control the urge to act out her angry feelings towards him. A similar dynamic existed between Mr M and his wife and one can hypothesise that Mr M's (unconscious) anger and resentment of his wife's increased power over him, and feelings of humiliation due to incontinence and decreased virility led to his rage that erupted in the very violent attack on his wife. Consideration of the differing feelings that Mr M evoked in different members of the staff looking after him led to an understanding of how splitting was occurring within the team, into which Mr M was projecting different parts of his internal object relationships. The team agreed that the risk of Mr M becoming violent again towards his wife should not be underestimated and couple therapy was recommended to facilitate Mr M and his wife in acknowledging the unconscious tensions between them.

Inadequate analysis of the clinician's emotional responses to the patient can contribute to faulty risk assessment that may in itself increase risk. For example, patients' actions can provoke anger, fear or disgust which may elicit punitive or sadistic responses in professionals, so that risk is overestimated and inappropriate interventions such as prolonged incarceration or physical restraint are instituted, which may not be necessary. The patient's subsequent anger and resentment at feeling punished and mistreated may lead to an increased risk of his behaving dangerously. Other offenders may elicit sympathy and present themselves as innocent victims who are not responsible for their actions, which may resonate with a clinician's "rescue fantasies" in their desire to treat patients whom they perceive have been misunderstood and mistreated by other professionals, so that the risk here is underestimated. Patients who minimize the seriousness of their offences, or who claim amnesia for the event, are often mistaken for deliberately lying or malingering, but their excessive use of defence mechanisms such as denial or amnesia may not be conscious. The inability to remember may be understood neurophysiologically as the person's mind being in too much of a state of arousal to be able to register their actions in retrievable memory, but can also be understood from a psychodynamic perspective in that remembering what has been done and fully acknowledging the consequences would mean feeling unbearable pain, guilt and loss. The presence of such amnesia, or the extensive use of other defence mechanisms such as denial or projection, however, should ring alarm bells when considering future risk.

Clinical example

Mr J was a 60-year-old man transferred from prison to a medium secure unit whilst awaiting sentencing for killing his second wife. He had been married for twenty years to a woman with intractable health problems. Mr J had a history of depression himself and had been his wife's main carer, but denied that there had been any difficulties or tensions between them. Mr J claimed he had no recollection of the killing except afterwards finding himself covered in blood and ringing the police saying he had done something terrible. His wife had been stabbed in the chest many times. On the ward Mr J did not appear depressed and could offer no explanation for the killing. He acknowledged that he must have killed his wife as he was the only other person there, but did not appear to fully own responsibility for his actions. The nurses found him quiet and co-operative.

His past medical records, however, revealed that 25 years earlier he had been convicted for another homicide—the murder of his first wife who had also had chronic health problems. This attack had also involved severe and frenzied violence.

The charge of murder was reduced to manslaughter on the basis of diminished responsibility, and Mr J was admitted to a low secure unit on a restricted order of the Mental Health Act (Section 37/41). He remained on the ward for several years and was described as a model patient. Significantly, he had no memory of this first killing either, and again described the relationship with his first wife as without conflict. He met his second wife whilst in hospital, and several

> years later he successfully applied for his restriction order to be rescinded.
>
> When asked about his history, Mr J denied any difficulties in his relationships with his parents, but did admit to having spent long periods of his childhood in hospital due to a bone disorder requiring corrective surgery. His parents had been very protective of him and his childhood had been rather isolated with few friends and disrupted schooling, but he did not see these as adverse experiences. He described himself as a quiet, peaceful man, perhaps prone to depression but not violence.

Here we can see the extreme split between Mr J's conscious experience of himself as a man who avoided conflicts, and his murderous rage, which is split off from consciousness and enacted in his very violent behaviour. This rage is inaccessible to Mr J's conscious mind, and it seems was also not acknowledged by those responsible for his care and follow-up in the community after the original killing. There did not appear to be concern that Mr J was forming a relationship with a woman who had very similar characteristics to his first wife, in that both women had severe disabilities, and in both relationships Mr J was the main carer. It is also remarkable how similar the murderous acts were, despite being separated by a period of 25 years during which Mr J showed no violence, in fact behaved like a "model citizen" to the point where he was considered of minimal risk. This can be seen as an example of Freud's compulsion to repeat (1920) in which the patient is obliged to repeat the repressed material as a contemporary experience or action instead of remembering it as something belonging to the past. One could speculate that Mr J's repressed rage from his infantile experiences of being hospitalized and overprotected by his parents is enacted in his violence towards a vulnerable hated deformed image of himself, that is projected into his disabled wives and has to be killed off. He has again ended up as a long-term patient on a ward, as he was following his first offence, a repetition of his childhood experience of prolonged in-patient admissions. Such an environment may be the one place in which he feels his violence can be contained.

Containment

Risk can only be managed safely if the anxieties of patients, individual staff and the institutions in which they work are adequately contained. "Containment" is a term originally introduced by Bion (1959, 1962) in describing the function of projective identification in the analytic situation as paralleling the way the baby projects its unbearable distress into the mother who "contains" it and responds by modifying the baby's anxieties by her "reverie". This is her capacity to understand through empathic identification with her baby, bear the intolerable anxieties, moderate them and feed them back to her baby in a form in which he can tolerate them, thus promoting healthy mental and physical development. The analyst's function is the same—he "contains" the patient's projections in a state of "reverie" and responds with appropriate interpretations. Similarly, Winnicott (1954) described the "holding" function of the analyst and of the analytic situation in providing an atmosphere in which the patient can feel safe and contained even when severe regression has occurred.

The provision of such a containing environment is of paramount importance, not just for the patient but for the clinicians and other staff involved in their care. In high secure conditions such as special hospitals, or in medium secure units, staff commonly report feeling physically safe due to the locked wards and high walls, but emotionally insecure as they are the recipients of all the projections of the dangerous and disturbed patients with whom they work, and they may need help in order to contain the anxieties provoked in them. As personal therapy is often not available, the role of supervision, consultation and the provision of support groups may be essential in providing a reflective forum in which the patient's pathology and behaviour and impact on the staff can be thought about. If the busy staff can be persuaded to have a regular protected time and space in which to think about patients, rather than act or react (for example, by filling in forms, managing the ward, or administering the medication) the rate of violent incidents by patients on the ward may actually decrease.

In today's inner cities, the most uncontained environments may in fact be the acute psychiatric wards. A recent major inquiry into the state of London's mental health services (King's Fund, 2003) revealed that despite the introduction of the National Service Framework for Mental Health, demand for acute inpatient beds for people with mental health problems remains under intense pressure. The report highlighted the high level of compulsory admissions, the increasing number of patients with a psychotic illness who are also substance misusers, and that wards remain in unsuitable buildings seen as unsafe and unattractive by staff and service users alike. There are severe staff shortages, and all of the nurses interviewed reported fearing for their personal safety at work at some time.

Nurses may have the most patient contact, but it is important to encourage all members of the multidisciplinary team to participate in reflective practice. Medically trained staff may be more comfortable with the medical model, with its emphasis on diagnostic categories, which they use as a defence against thinking about patients as individuals who might have an emotional impact on them. The psychiatric trainee's lexicon is limited by a psychiatric classification system based on descriptive phenomenology, and which promotes a nosology with an officious vocabulary of "operational definitions" and "multi-axial criteria" which fails to obscure that this is now phenomenology removed from any meaning.

Clinical example

A case discussion group was run by an experienced psychotherapist for a group of junior psychiatrists, to discuss the patients they were involved in looking after in a variety of acute psychiatric settings. Dr B told the group about a case that had been troubling him. A 26-year-old man had been admitted recently and was under his care in the Intensive Care Unit. The man had initially presented to casualty several months previously, complaining that he had suffered a needle stick injury and he was afraid he had been infected with HIV. The patient could not give a reliable account of what had happened but said that someone had stabbed him in the street. Different versions of this story were given by the patient over the next few weeks during which he presented to the Accident and Emergency on several further occasions in an acute crisis, convinced he was HIV positive and feeling suicidal. He was eventually admitted to a general psychiatric ward, but his behaviour rapidly became aggressive and he was transferred to the Intensive Care Unit. The provisional diagnosis was delusional disorder, but the only apparent psychotic symptom he had was the delusion that he was HIV positive. Dr B felt incompetent in not knowing how to manage the violent behaviour of this man, who was uncooperative with treatment and had had to be forcibly injected with tranquillisers and anti-psychotic medication.

The psychotherapist facilitating the group asked if he could say more about the patient. He was the only son in a close family, and he had a particularly close relationship with his mother. His childhood and teenage years were described as entirely "normal" and after gaining A' levels he had worked for some years in regular employment with good prospects. It was felt that his personality was entirely "normal" and that he had never suffered any psychological or mental health difficulties previously. In passing it was briefly mentioned that his girlfriend of some years had become pregnant. The psychotherapist drew attention to this and asked when. The baby was due any day, and working backwards, Dr B worked out that the girl must have become pregnant shortly before the patient had first presented. However, little was known about what was happening to the girlfriend and baby now because the patient refused to talk about it. It appeared that the patient's attempt to obliterate this part of his life had led to the collusion of those involved in his care in participating in his denial, the imminent real baby had been forgotten and had been replaced by the patient.

The psychotherapist drew attention to the timing of the baby's conception which seemed to occur just before the putative needle-stick injury and suggested that the patient had unconsciously reversed the experience of an active penetration resulting in a pregnancy, so that he was the one who felt penetrated and infected with a fatal illness. She suggested that the patient's uncooperative and violent behaviour represented a regression to an earlier psycho-developmental stage, which had the result of him receiving 24-hour care and attention. The other doctors became interested, and another doctor who had also been involved in his care on the ward reported that the patient had tantrums like a toddler, and his mother and sisters visited daily bringing home-cooked food, and telling the staff he needed to be treated very gently. The psychotherapist suggested that to escape from feelings of jealousy and aggression towards the real baby whom he feared would replace him in his girlfriend's mind, he had regressed to being the baby again of his mother and sisters. With little psychological or systemic understanding of his "psychosis", the real baby had been forgotten, and the patient was fast on his way to a diagnosis of schizophrenia. The junior doctors reported that once a patient was admitted to the Intensive Care Ward, he could not avoid being treated with anti-psychotic medication and would usually have to be restrained. The psychotherapist suggested that whatever this man's diagnosis, involvement of the family would be likely to assist in his management and rehabilitation and reduce risk.

These junior doctors are working in an environment in which there is little time or space for thought, and the terror of the patient becomes actualized in violent behaviour, evoking a punitive response by staff in restraint, forcible injection or isolation, increasing risk to patients and staff alike. Such case-discussion groups run on Balint-style lines are now a required part of the training of junior psychiatrists, to facilitate the trainees in acquiring basic psychotherapeutic skills and concepts, such as the importance of the therapeutic alliance in the doctor–patient relationship, the significance of the psychiatrist's own feelings in any clinical situations, the psychodynamic formulation and the necessity of providing a safe setting in which neither psychiatrist nor patient feels at risk.

Confidentiality

Finally, I wish to consider how the communication of information regarding risk can affect the overall process of risk management. All clinicians have a duty of care to their patients in treating the communications between them as confidential. Such a duty is enshrined in professional codes of conduct, such as the age-old physician's Hippocratic oath, or the more recent General Medical Council's guidelines on confidentiality (2004). Some (e.g. Bollas and Sundelson, 1995) may argue that confidentiality in the therapeutic situation should be preserved unconditionally, whilst a more pragmatic view is that disclosure of information to other parties is necessary under special circumstances where there is risk of serious harm to the patient or others. For a patient to engage in a therapeutic process he needs to feel that he can trust the therapist with thoughts, fantasies and feelings that he may be ashamed or terrified of admitting to himself, let alone others. The therapist treads a delicate balance in cultivating a gradual awareness in the patient's mind of such previously repressed fantasies and anxieties without being perceived by the patient as orchestrating a violent assault on his internal world. This process is facilitated by the therapist creating a safe and containing environment within the boundaries of the therapeutic relationship, boundaries that include the concrete reliability of the physical environment in which the therapy takes place, as well as the interpersonal boundaries between patient and therapist, in which the therapist minimizes self-disclosure as well as the disclosure of the contents of the therapy to others.

However, there may be some circumstances in which not to disclose information to others may be detrimental to the patient. The therapist's decision to alert others to a possible increased risk posed by the patient may be felt by the patient as being understood and taken seriously, and such disclosure in itself may decrease risk. By contrast, if the therapist opts not to disclose worrying fantasies or behaviour that have emerged in the therapy, the patient may feel as if he has fooled the therapist, or that the therapist is colluding in something dangerous, and therefore cannot be trusted. The patient should be encouraged to make any disclosures himself, which can lead to a greater sense of responsibility for his actions. The involvement of a real third object, who can intervene in the patient therapist dyad, can create a triangular situation in which a different point of view can be considered, and the patient himself can feel understood and contained by a more healthy parental couple.

Clinical example

A 35-year-old man Mr A was being seen in weekly individual therapy by a female therapist. He had been brought up by a single mother, who had physically abused him, and as an adolescent he had made several serious suicide attempts. He was married but described a sado-masochistic relationship with his wife whom he experienced as humiliating and castrating, but allowed her to offer her services as a prostitute to other men. A sado-masochistic dynamic was quickly established in the transference, with Mr A spending most sessions verbally attacking and belittling the therapist such that she felt her therapeutic skills were undermined and dreaded seeing him. Mr A would tell her how incompetent she was compared to the much more experienced male psychiatrist whose care he had been under for many years.

Prior to the therapist's annual leave over Christmas, Mr A reported feeling suicidal, and the therapist was also concerned for the welfare of his 13-year-old daughter, for whom he was the main carer. He had recently allowed her to visit the flat of a neighbour, who was a registered sex offender. The patient taunted the therapist with an account of his most recent appointment with his psychiatrist who had apparently claimed not to know the therapist's name, meaning that she must be very junior and perhaps unqualified to help him. He admitted, however, feeling "fobbed off" by the psychiatrist, who had not wanted to see him again for six months. With the agreement of the patient, the therapist decided to contact the psychiatrist to voice her concerns about how he would cope during the forthcoming break. The therapist and psychiatrist met and the psychiatrist agreed to see the patient during the therapist's absence. After the therapy resumed, the patient admitted how he felt he had been cared for by both the professionals involved in his care, had not felt like harming himself during the break and had arranged for some extra help in looking after his daughter. Here, the therapist's disclosures resulted in Mr A feeling that his anxieties had been understood by a parental couple that could work together in his best interests, unlike the real parental couple of his childhood, and the risk of harm both to Mr A and to his daughter was reduced.

Conclusion

For better or for worse, decision-making regarding risk and dangerousness is inescapable for all those working within the field of mental health today and forms a fundamental influence on clinical practice and mental health policy. It is important that such considerations can be thought about before being acted upon, and I hope I have shown how a psychoanalytic approach can contribute to this process. Such an approach can transform routine risk assessment and management from being a sterile formulaic exercise that may be resented, to one that is meaningful to the individual patient and his history. Central to this is the recognition of the unconscious communications that exist, expressed in the behaviour of the dangerous patient, and in the counter-transferential responses of all those involved in the patient's care and management. The real risk is of categorizing a patient as dangerous due to a predetermined set of criteria, before considering each patient as an individual with his own unique history that has influenced his thoughts, feelings and behaviours in multi-determined fashion. Adequate risk assessment can only be achieved through real patient contact, by prioritizing the development of a therapeutic relationship between patient and clinician, whether the latter be doctor, nurse, social worker or psychotherapist. Awareness of the unconscious communications and defence mechanisms operating within the mental health team or institution will promote effective communication and the provision of a containing environment that is necessary to manage risk safely.

Finally, one should not forget the dangers of developing omnipotent or complacent attitudes. Risk can be reduced but never eliminated, and mistakes and tragedies will inevitably occur. We must resist the increasing tendency of society to blame individual clinicians for the actions of their patients, which can be so damaging for the morale of all those dedicated to working in the very rewarding but challenging arena of mental health.

CHAPTER FIVE

Psychoanalytical aspects to the risk of containment of dangerous patients treated in high security

Carine Minne

The perplexing or shocking behaviours that can lead patients, psychotic or otherwise, to be treated in secure settings under the care of forensic psychiatry teams may have contributed to those clinical teams in particular incorporating a psychoanalytic approach. Another reason for this might be that a psychoanalytic approach is considered helpful with those patients suffering from personality disorders for whom the "ordinary" psychiatric management does not seem to suffice. In this chapter, I will first describe in a general way how clinical psychiatric teams in high secure hospital settings approach the problem of patients who have been violent. I will then give examples of "dangerous" patients who have been treated with psychoanalytic psychotherapy and show how this approach can contribute to understanding their difficulties and violent propensities, adding an important aspect to their management.

Patients looked after in Special Hospital or high security are, by virtue of having been sent there, considered to be dangerous. To be dangerous is generally used to mean that a particular individual, based on previous violent acts by that person, is likely to behave violently again. Violence in psychiatric literature is widely accepted to be "the intended infliction of bodily harm on another person" and this definition requires there to be a breach in body boundary (Glasser, 1979a, 1985). The first difficulty immediately apparent in attempting to examine the problem of dangerousness in a patient from a psychoanalytical perspective is that the description refers to the quality of an individual's previous actions rather than saying anything about the individual himself (Mullen, 1984). This causes a pull towards a behavioural approach in examining the problem because violent acts can be seen and measured. This approach alone does not suffice and the simple fact that a previously violent person has not been violent for a certain amount of time, which could be years, does not tell us anything about the likelihood of future violent behaviour. Neither does it provide any understanding or meaning of the violence committed. A multi-factorial perspective is necessary in order to have meaningful clinical appraisals. A psychoanalytic approach can contribute by offering a view of such a patient's mind and in what way his or her past dangerous behaviour resides in that mind. Psychoanalytic theories are useful in the quest to understand why certain patients suffering from mental disorders and who have carried out serious violence acts, appear to have inadequate defences against the discharge of violent impulses. One should not forget that, amidst the near pathognomonic presence of environmental contributing factors, constitutional features might also play a role.

A history of previous violence is considered as the best predictor of future violence for all people, mentally disordered or not. To simply keep patients in high security locked up indefinitely, apart from being unethical, ignores the multi-faceted nature of dangerousness, the temporal dimension and the existence of treatments that can be offered to those with mental disorders. It also implies that society might believe it can rid itself of a problem or even that only revenge matters and if there is any hope of change with treatments that can be offered, these are not deserved. These are the primitive "tabloid" ways of dealing with these complex issues which are inhumane, short-sighted and, just like the problem behaviours these patients present with, mindless. One task for the clinical team looking after these patients and, perhaps in particular, the psychoanalytic psychotherapist, is to help them begin to "mind" what they have had to keep "mindless". Nevertheless, It is important to bear in mind the role of public perception of mentally disordered offenders and how this influences policy makers, particularly those involved with the high secure hospital patient population. It could be considered an ethical obligation of those professionals involved in treating this patient population to have an input in policy-making.

The three Special Hospitals in England and Wales (Broadmoor, Rampton and Ashworth) provide psychiatric care under conditions of high security for patients who must *pose a grave and immediate risk.* These hospitals house approximately one and a half thousand patients who are detained under the 1983 Mental Health Act (mainly under sections in part 3 of that Act which deals with patients concerned in criminal proceedings or sentences), which is under review since the Mental Health White Paper (December 2000). The second part of this White Paper addressed the "High Risk Patients" and outlined new criteria that would link compulsory powers with treatment plans needed to treat mental disorders or manage behaviours arising from the disorders. This part of the White Paper also referred to the establishment of new facilities for those who are dangerous and severely personality disordered (DSPD) and about which there remains some controversy.

Most patients in high security are considered dangerous some of the time and only when certain ingredients come together. It is another task of the clinical team who look after such patients to continuously review these ingredients or factors and the totality of this is now referred to as "risk containment" (Monahan, 1993). This is a term used to describe the multifaceted approach required when considering a patient who has been dangerous. Snowden (1997) has provided a helpful way of considering risk containment under three broad headings.

Firstly, that of risk identification. In other words, what is the risk being considered? Is it a risk of harm towards the self or of behaving violently towards others? Is the risk one of relapse of a particular mental illness that is known to be associated with violent behaviour?

Secondly, once the risk is identified, one assesses that risk in terms of frequency with which it might recur and the severity of any recurrence. In addition to actuarial risk assessment, as much information as possible should be obtained about the patient's background and past, including previous and present behaviour as well as previous and present mental states. All possible sources of information should be sought by the different professionals in the clinical team, ranging from obtaining old school reports, to speaking with relatives or neighbours or examining police records or social work reports. This enables a thorough appraisal of as many facets as possible of a particular patient, leading to the best-informed clinical judgement that can be made in assessing the risk. Risk is something that varies over time and therefore has to be constantly reappraised.

The third heading is that of clinical risk management and is about treating the patient's mental disorder by providing the patient with multi-disciplinary input that helps reduce the frequency and severity of the identified and assessed risks. One form of treatment, directly or indirectly applied, is psychoanalytic psychotherapy. A long-term aim is to enable patients to "contain" themselves.

Looking at it from the perspective of the whole institution, risk containment such as described above for each individual case, should be systematically reviewed and revised with regular clinical auditing and research. Risk containment can then, hopefully, become more refined and continue to develop to benefit patients, those looking after them and society. All these aspects of a patient's management also form part of the wider rubric of the Care Programme Approach that must be applied to every patient suffering from mental disorder to ensure that they get the full care and support they need once back in the community.

The level of dangerousness of any patient in high secure conditions such as these is a matter that has to be assessed repeatedly for good clinical monitoring of the patients. This is to ensure that they receive the most effective treatments available, and that the appropriate level of observation is provided by nursing staff so that they can ensure the safety of staff and patients. This is something that can vary from day to day. Such regular monitoring also helps ensure that the patients are placed in the appropriate level of security and that, when ready to move to less secure conditions, this is judged thoughtfully on clinical grounds.

How does somebody become a Special Hospital patient? The patients in high security come directly from the courts when a hospital order has been imposed on them, or they may be transferred from prison whilst on remand for assessment or treatment, or if they have become ill whilst serving a sentence. They may also be transferred from less secure hospital conditions if managing them there has become problematic. It is certainly worth bearing in mind that approximately one third of the sentenced prison population of

England and Wales (now over 75,000) is estimated to suffer from some kind of mental disorder (Gunn & Maden, 1991) and that several hundred of these people require treatment in a secure hospital which cannot be provided to the extent needed because of shortage of secure hospital facilities. It is mainly long stay medium secure hospital beds that are desperately needed.

It is a frequent misperception that people in high secure hospital conditions are referred to as prisoners or inmates. They have certainly lost their freedom but they are patients in hospital to receive treatment. The pull to calling them prisoners is the familiar pull towards a custodial and punitive focus and away from the idea of treatment, often misconstrued by the general public as condoning the awful offences that have been committed. What is required is the right balance for each individual case between the positions of treatment, provided by the mental health professionals, and punishment plus loss of freedom, provided respectively by the Criminal Justice System and the secure environment, both essential for the proper care of any patient and the safety of the public. The difficulties in achieving this balance contribute to one of the particular dynamics when working under conditions of high security where providing treatment and security can seem to clash.

For example, all those working in Special Hospital carry, tied to their waists, an enormous bunch of keys and the impact of this cannot be ignored, simply in terms of adding to the "them" versus "us" scenario, or "envious" versus "enviable". Here, straight away, a most concrete split is set up which could almost be described as those present, patients and professionals, being dressed in their respective costumes ready to enact the familiar sado-masochistic script so often apparent in situations where dangerous or "bad" people are housed. Unless one remains constantly aware of this, one can easily fall prey to the magnetic pull of such transference and counter-transference phenomena and realize again and again the patients' internal worlds for them that they can succeed in getting the professionals to sculpt with them. In such institutions, primitive psychodynamics fly around in all directions when patients with these levels of disturbance are brought together with their special expertise of projecting all over the place and inside every available container, mainly the nurses. They have the most difficult task of all in these hospitals, being the main recipients of these projections as they are with the patients 24 hours a day. This, in turn, places the nurses in one of the most valuable positions in terms of monitoring the patients' states of minds, and hence contributing towards the assessment of dangerousness which, as stated earlier, needs to be a continuous part of the risk containment of these patients.

How can a forensic psychoanalytic psychotherapist come into the picture and offer another dimension towards making the best risk containment strategy for any given patient? This can be by working directly with patients in therapy, which offers an opportunity for regular reviewing of patients' mental states whilst working therapeutically. Alternatively, by working indirectly, through supervising other professionals treating these patients in therapy, or by being available to speak to primary nurses (each patient is allocated his or her own main or primary nurse) about their patients in the hope of offering them another way of speaking and listening to their patients. Attending ward rounds and case conferences where patients' management is discussed is also a forum where the presence of the forensic psychoanalytic psychotherapist can be useful, for example by helping a team that might have become divided about how a particular patient should best be managed. The aim in all of these situations is to improve the awareness of the unconscious processes at work. An awareness of the unconscious processes of a patient's mind and consequently, of his or her interactions, can add an invaluable dimension to risk assessment. Providing psychoanalytic therapeutic treatment as part of the overall care plan, or clinical risk management, can also contribute to the "risk containment" of a particular case.

It is one major task of this kind of psychotherapy to enable awareness of the mind and its functions to become available to the owner of that mind, the patient. This refers to an awareness of who they are, what they have done and the impact of this on their minds and on the minds of others, i.e. making what is unconscious, conscious. Often, patients who have carried out serious violent offences demonstrate a high degree of unawareness, regardless of their diagnosis. This can manifest itself in various ways such as denial, disavowal, minimization, amnesia, to name but a few mechanisms. One could say that this lack of awareness can appear to be necessary for the patient's psychic survival. This is an unfortunate situation where the risk of the patient acting dangerously again remains unchanged.

The alternative to "not knowing" could be to become overwhelmed by the knowledge of who they are and what they have done. This can cause massive anxieties about "cracking up" and can lead to psychotic breakdowns (if they are not already manifestly psychiatrically psychotic) and, perhaps, to suicide. The therapist's task is a delicate and complicated one; how to help the cultivation of awareness in the patient's mind without seeming to commit a violent assault to that person's mind. Secondly, how to clinically judge that such awareness is developing and, thirdly, in what way is it being used by the patient? Experience has shown that any such achievements by a patient and therapist together can function, at an unconscious level, as a provocation of a part of the patient's mind that envies what the union of patient and therapist have managed together and wants this destroyed, achieving this through denigration of the work done.

A difficult balance to achieve, as a psychotherapist working in these situations, is that of confidentiality to the patient versus the need to communicate information if and when security or risk issues arise. This is something that has to be reviewed every time an issue of this kind comes up. As a psychoanalytic psychotherapist, one tries to offer patients confidentiality for obvious therapeutic reasons. One might perhaps facilitate a patient's informing of the clinical team of a change in risk, for example, in dangerousness towards self or another. This is sometimes not possible and then one has to assess how best to proceed. This may result in a need to communicate something to the clinical team although this should be discussed with the patient. I have found that patients are often relieved to be helped inform the team of a change in risk, or relieved if I do this for them, even though their getting me to "do" something has then to be interpreted. The procedure of patient, or therapist on behalf of patient, disclosing can itself result in a diminution of the risk being communicated by virtue of the patient having felt to be understood. This is one of the striking differences between forensic psychotherapy and psychotherapy generally, that of the presence of a real third object, or a triangular situation (Welldon, 1994).

I shall try to illustrate this way of working using some (anonymized and altered for reasons of confidentiality) examples of patients looked after in high security hospitals who have had psychoanalytic psychotherapy as part of their treatment plan. There are, of course, many other examples of patients who have not had individual psychoanalytic psychotherapy but where a psychoanalytic approach has also been used in assessing and treating. This is more often the case in high security patients where only a few can be offered individual therapy of this kind at present. Many more patients are treated in psychoanalytical psychotherapy groups. The clinical teams also use psychoanalytically informed thinking or consultation in order to provide a consistent, unified approach to their patients, which avoids unconsciously colluding with aspects of their psychopathology.

Case study one

Mr A is 24 years old and was admitted to a high secure hospital when a court imposed a hospital order with a Home Office restriction at the conclusion of his trial. He had been convicted of murder. The offence for which he was arrested occurred in a public place late one evening when no one other than his female victim was around. He carried out what appeared to be an impulsive unprovoked and extremely serious attack on a woman using a sharp weapon, leaving her fatally injured and running away before giving himself up to the police. He had no prior record of violent offences. He did not appear overtly mentally disordered but his vulnerability and neediness were soon detected whilst he was on remand in prison and this, combined with his young age, led to psychiatric reports being requested for his trial.

At first, Mr A's offence was described by him as a one-off event, a handbag theft that had gone wrong. However, the extreme violence that he had used, which was to attack this woman with the full strength of his body, was not in keeping with this explanation and it was considered early on that psychically, a different scenario might have been acted out. After several months in hospital, he admitted this. This was a conscious withholding on his part of what he thought he knew of what he was doing at the time of the offence as opposed to any unconscious denial.

He started twice-weekly psychoanalytic psychotherapy shortly after his admission to high security. He pleaded to have this and as soon as it was offered, began to use the sessions to complain about how little this was compared with what he needed. He said that he wanted and should have someone available to talk to 24 hours a day, someone who would provide continuous unconditional care. His mother had in fact left the family home with a lover when his younger sibling was born, leaving her husband to look after a 3-year-old toddler, Mr A, and a new-born baby. It was not difficult to piece together that, as a very young child, Mr A had suffered a major trauma, one of unprocessed grief of an enormous early loss. This loss, perhaps in combination with his particular constitution, must have caused his mind to fill with unbearable feelings of rage he had to get rid of. Around the age of 4 years, he began to make plasticine models with a violent content—figurines attacking each other with weapons. This was apparently a preoccupation beyond the ordinary limits of any little boy's play. He also started to behave aggressively towards little children who seemed to have "nice mummies" bringing them to school. These may have been early manifestations of a very troubled child, furiously unhappy at being abandoned by his mother, the cause appearing to be the arrival of a baby girl who displaced not only him but also his mother. He also may have experienced envious feelings regarding those who seemed to have what he so desperately wanted, a "nice mummy". Sadly, these early manifestations of his disturbance, that were in fact noticed by parental figures and teachers, were addressed unhelpfully by simply being reprimanded for making and doing ugly things.

With the onset of puberty, Mr A's unresolved rage became attached to his developing sexual feelings. He began to masturbate to fantasies of rape and strangulation. This evolved into stalking women and, several times, he came close to attacking a particular woman he had been following, only to "chicken out" at the last moment, leaving the woman totally unaware of what had nearly happened to her. The victim was not so fortunate. Initially, what he presented as a robbery that went wrong could later be seen in quite a different light, an apparently impulsive attack that was actually one that had been premeditated and rehearsed over a long period of time. There had also been the ominous development of an escalation in his dangerousness from fantasy only, to practising carrying these out, and finally, an incomplete enactment of his main fantasy. Here we can see how the capacity to symbolise (through fantasies) gradually breaks down as the severity of the psychotic functioning increases, leading to the need to act out. Anxiety is engendered by the very fantasies that are created in order to resolve it. This fuels the escalation until the fantasies no longer suffice and deterioration into action is required.

This is a young man whose toddler and probably infantile feelings of rage at the loss of his mother threaten to overwhelm his psyche. He therefore has to get rid of these in the only way he can, by projecting them violently into a recipient who fulfils his unconscious criteria.

Any woman can be a potential victim of his if she is experienced by him to ignore him and to behave as if nothing is the matter. His female victim, who turned away from facing him, could be said to represent the mother who turns her back on him as well as being a woman who is free of the disturbance he is experiencing. This patient envies the capacity of his objects, or women, to be immune to the disease he is full of. The female victim was also someone who, in his mind, is happily on her way home and therefore has a home to go to which he does not. At that moment (of perceiving the woman to be ignoring him and happily going home), he has to defend against the rage and anxiety that his states of motherlessness and homelessness provoke in him and which he feels at that moment have been provoked by the object, the woman aggressor. He tries to achieve this by reversing the situation of feeling at the mercy of a cruel and abandoning object, and instead attempting to control the object by the rape, which did not happen (but would have been another way of filling the object with his rage) and the killing, which did. One could say that it was not her handbag he was trying to steal but her sense of well-being.

In his therapy, he tries to defend against the perceived attacks on his psyche by presenting himself as knowing exactly what he needs and should have and demanding these. He cannot be satiated. When he experiences the inevitable frustrations of his unmet demands, or when he discovers that he is not in control of his objects, he becomes furious. This can be triggered by, for example, the therapist saying that the session has ended. The loss of his omnipotently created control of his object leads to a fury that knows no other way of being experienced other than to get rid of it by acting it violently, hence the need to take special precautions to provide safety for patient and therapist around the sessions. This fury was confirmed by the patient who described feeling like a pressure cooker inside his head, and how that pressure was released in the split second following the attack.

This situation can also be repeated in his therapy when he occasionally hears what he has not decided I should say to him, in other words, when, once more, I am not what and how he wants me to be. His response in these moments can either be one of furore, when he shouts angrily at me or walks out before "losing it" or, alternatively, he experiences being the victim of my psychic assault on his mind. During these moments, Mr A is highly dangerous. In the first situation, his propensity to act violently towards me or somebody else on the ward is massively increased momentarily, or at least until that particular state of mind subsides. In the second situation, the risk of dangerousness is greater against himself when he might deliberately harm himself whilst he feels himself to be the victim, not just of his therapist but of the whole awful world he then wants to punish by inducing guilt. He can be simultaneously identified with both aggressor and victim. The experience of being his therapist is that one can be made to feel very anxious and frightened at those intense moments and it is important to use those feelings constructively to formulate the best interpretation under the difficult circumstances. It is vital to acknowledge one's fear to oneself as well as to use this to speak to the patient informatively about what he is then doing to you, his object.

Occasionally, this particular patient presents as innocent and harmless, as a nice young man. At these moments, the patient is actually sufficiently disturbed to believe his delusion of being a nice young man who is misunderstood. It is my view that, at these moments, the patient's belief is of delusional intensity and not simply an overvalued idea. This presentation can be very convincing as well as alluring, and professionals can find it hard not to be taken in. One way of trying to avoid feeling anxious and frightened whilst being with such a patient is to collude with their delusion of not being disturbed. Serious errors of judgement can be made at these moments. To reassure the patient at this moment might well serve as a sedative for both patient and therapist but is a false reassurance for both. These "nice" states are often brittle and can swiftly shift to a more obvious hostile presentation or angry state of mind. For example, this patient has been known to shout at me, "How can you say that? You treat me as if I was a dangerous person." At this moment, the patient's awareness of who he is and what he has done is not available to him and the therapist, in order to be of any use to the patient at that moment, has to be prepared to remind the patient of what he definitely does not want to be reminded of. This interpretation can be experienced by the patient as an attempt by the therapist to kill him, albeit psychically, which he may need to defend himself against, again a moment of increased risk of dangerousness when he might get rid of his feelings by acting them out. The next immediate interpretation therefore needs to be to show the patient how, when he is reminded of who he is, he feels traumatized by this. The hope is that when this has been repeated in therapy hundreds of times, each time it may become less necessary for this to be a bodily experience of rage and terror by the patient and more able to be experienced in his mind. These moments of increased risk of acting out by the patient are diminished in frequency and intensity by the constant working through of the repetitious splits that take place. The therapeutic work attempts to transform the patient from having no awareness of himself and being obliviously at risk of again behaving dangerously, to having awareness of himself and being mentally equipped to be able to deal with the traumatic effect of this knowledge and the despair it can cause.

Case study two

Ms B is a 27-year-old woman who killed her 9-week-old daughter and later, seriously wounded a professional. She comes from a large and highly dysfunctional family where trans-generational incestuous relationships have resulted in no one being sure of who is who in the extended family. Violence between different sets of parents, mother with father and mother with stepfathers, was the norm. There was no experience of consistent mothering. This young woman developed a tic disorder around puberty that was eventually treated with medication. She met a young man when she was 19 years old and made a conscious decision that he was the man she would leave home for, marry, and have children with. Prior to this, she had no serious boyfriends and one could speculate to what extent Ms B was attempting to undo some of the chaos she had been raised in by having a "white wedding". She and her husband lived together with his alcoholic mother following their marriage.

Ms B was soon delighted to discover she was pregnant. However, the stress of this event on an ill-equipped young couple like this, led to the breakdown of their marriage late in her pregnancy when she returned home to live with her own mother. Within days of delivering a healthy baby girl, her mother asked her to leave and go to live elsewhere. This was quite typical behaviour of this mother who later, for example, frequently told the patient, her daughter, that she probably would be better off committing suicide than causing all this trouble. Ms B and her newborn baby moved in with a family friend.

Ms B developed concerns about her baby soon after she was born. She was convinced that the baby was sick and called her Health Visitor and General Practitioner on a regular basis but could never accept reassurance. On one occasion, she stated that the baby had started to manifest facial tics like her own, of such severity that the baby's breathing was affected. The mother and baby were admitted to hospital for the baby to be monitored. Initially, the baby was found to be well but after two days, the baby's condition began to deteriorate. No cause for this deterioration could be found. The baby became critically ill and needed to be looked after in intensive care before dying from cardiac and respiratory failure that did not respond to intensive treatment.

Ms B, bereft, went home with her mother. Soon after the baby's death and post-mortem, laboratory reports showed toxic levels of a particular medication in the baby's blood that were considered to have caused the death from poisoning. This was the medication Ms B was on for her illness. She was arrested and charged with murdering her baby. In view of her fragile mental state, her remand period was spent in a psychiatric hospital. She denied any wrong doing for over a year, until the end of the trial, when she admitted having given the baby her medication, not to kill the baby but out of concern that the doctors and nurses were not looking after the baby properly. Retrospectively, it could be suggested that she projected her own bad experience of being mothered twice over, once into her own baby, by identifying with her mother and then again, by projective identification with the nurses and doctors, who became the bad parents for not noticing what was going on within the sick baby, herself, as well as the actual sick baby.

Ms B was admitted to medium security on a hospital order from the court, having been finally convicted of manslaughter. She had to be transferred to high security after seriously wounding a member of staff. She had also become violent towards herself, cutting herself deeply, hanging herself and making attempts to strangle herself.

Ms B started in twice-weekly psychoanalytic psychotherapy following her transfer to high security. During the first few months of treatment, she presented as a model, compliant patient who did as she imagined was expected of her in that situation which is no more than one can expect from someone with such a history. I mean that she presented as a distressed patient who spoke about what a dreadful thing she had done but all of this had a pseudo-feel to it. This way of presenting to me was gradually shown to her and interpreted as one way she had of avoiding feeling traumatized or victimized by her own disturbed state of mind at the time of her offences and now, in the room with me. This led to suicidality and a further increase in her dangerousness towards herself for a period of time.

In some sessions during these early months of therapy, she was more able to speak to me about what she did to her baby, how she crushed her tablets and secretly fed this to the baby, over and over again. At these moments, her real distress was very apparent. She described her preoccupation at the time with her belief that the baby was not being looked after properly by the nurses and doctors. I said to her, at these moments in her sessions, how she wished to be the baby that could be looked after properly. This is a highly ambivalent situation for this patient where she is faced with the problem that to be looked after properly negates her view of what proper looking after within her family structure means, creating a sense of betraying her family if she follows the trend of her therapy. I had to be kept, therefore, as someone who was bound to harm her in some way, and her history and offence were once more re-enacted.

The pathological mother-child dynamic present in this patient's mind could also be seen in her therapy when, unbeknown to anyone, she took an overdose before a session and then came for her therapy appearing with glazed eyes and bilateral hand tremor. She denied several times that anything was the matter when her physical state was commented on, before becoming angry and shouting that there was no point in all this, she wanted to be with her baby, another reference to her suicidality. She kept me in a concerned state and, after considering the likelihood of her having taken an overdose (because of a particular constellation of symptoms that became more apparent), I told her that I thought she wanted me to be a good mother and guess what was the matter. This was followed by a long silence. I then said that I believed she would be relieved if I guessed. I proceeded to tell her that I thought she wanted me to know that she had taken an overdose. If I did not notice this, then she could congratulate herself that she was right, no one notices she is serious (about suicide). If I did notice, she would get something from me but it would feel spoilt because of how she got it. In this situation, the patient did finally admit to having taken an overdose which then had to be urgently dealt with, medically. Again, in this session, the offence is repeated, a baby, herself, is harmed, again with medication, but this time the baby is saved. Indeed, the "being saved" actually led to a manic outburst of profuse thanks from the patient, diluting the seriousness of what had just happened and avoiding the experience of guilt that such a saving could provoke. For this patient, to commit suicide could also be seen as a re-enactment of her offence by killing her mother's baby.

During the second and third years of treatment, the patient's mental state gradually altered, vacillating between states of manic well-being, when she would deny any need of further treatment, and overt hostility towards her therapist who would not collude with her delusion of wellness. The periods of hostility were occasionally very severe and lasting many months. At these times, her dangerousness towards her therapist was judged to be high and special precautions had to be taken. This was a patient who had seriously wounded a member of staff who once told her to put away all the photographs she clung on to of her baby, that it was now time to get on with her life. The patient, at that moment, may have perceived that person as telling her to bring to an end her apparent mourning. Again, this is a complicated situation for Ms B where the nature of the attachment to the object that has been harmed, the baby, has to be questioned and consequently, so too must the nature of the mourning. During the periods of overt hostility towards her therapist, the patient may have perceived the therapist as telling her to continue with the apparent mourning when she wanted to be manically freed of this. Neither of these is a satisfactory position for Ms B's unresolved and complicated bereaved state. The patient is a danger to those intimately involved with her at those moments, her therapist, main nurses and other professionals closely involved in her care (also certain patients on the same ward who are known to take on "co-therapist" roles), rather than posing a risk to strangers.

Late in the third year of treatment, Ms B's mental state deteriorated into a more overtly psychotic presentation when she appeared perplexed and had paranoid delusions of being poisoned by staff as well as experiencing olfactory and auditory hallucinations. She stopped eating and drinking and required transfer to the medical ward where she seemed relieved and gratified from being tube fed, which she never refused, as though delegating her need to torture herself to those around her, including her therapist. What emerged from this more psychotic presentation several months later was a patient who appeared to be depressed and who described suffering a very low mood. She also presented with many of the biological symptoms of depression as well as prominent psychomotor retardation. She complained of flashbacks and nightmares, the content of these always being about her daughter's last hours attached to life-saving equipment and then in the morgue with a damaged dead body. Many sessions were brief and consisted of the patient slowly shuffling into the room reporting the following with her head down, no eye contact and in a monotonous voice; "I can't keep going like this, I want to be with my baby, I can't continue with this therapy, I can't stand the pain, I don't deserve to live, I don't deserve to die, look what I did to my baby, I must suffer for this". She would eventually ask a nurse to come and liberate her from me. I would try to take up with her how she mercilessly punished the baby's mother, herself. I would also take up with her how I was felt to be the punitive one, punishing the baby's mother. She was the baby as well, being harmed by me and who needed to be rescued from me by the nurses. The patient could be described here as having changed into a more Post Traumatic Stress Disorder *type* of presentation. There appears to be a clash in her mind between

> the part that killed her baby and knows it, colliding with the grieving part that experiences the flashbacks and that longs to be an ordinary grieving mother. A main struggle at this time in the therapy was whether she could face up to knowing who she was and what she had done and therefore be able to change, or whether she preferred to go back to, or stay in, a state of not knowing. In my view, there is a link between these positions in terms of her dangerousness. In the situation of not knowing herself and remaining unaware, she remains a chronic risk to her babies, actual ones or symbolic representations of them. The pathological mother-child dynamic remains intact. In the situation of getting to know herself and being helped to deal with this knowledge, the risk to these babies diminishes but, without treatment, or good risk management, the risk of dangerousness to herself rises.

The aim in providing therapy to these patients in this way, as part of the overall treatment, is to attempt to bring about a gradual realization of themselves, what they have done and what kind of mental life they lived before that allowed these awful events. These previous mental lives or mental states are those that the patients resume when in regressed states. The process of treatment appears to require a complicated and lengthy transition period from not knowing anything about themselves to becoming aware and dealing with the profoundly traumatic effects of this. The hope is to help them gain understanding and, optimistically, some change in their internal worlds. This may mean a change in presentation from a more pathologically defended personality disordered or psychotic presentation to one reminiscent of a Post Traumatic Stress Disorder presentation where the patient might feel early on, much worse, more distressed but would have, hopefully, a healthier internal world. This would be one where thoughts and feelings about what happened and their predicament in relation to this could be experienced in mind without the need to get rid of these in the familiar ways of acting them out violently. It is a lot to ask from people who suffer triple traumas, first of their unfortunate background histories, secondly, that of discovering themselves to have a mental disorder and thirdly, the trauma of having to deal with the serious violent offences they commit and the impact of these on others and themselves. I believe that this psychoanalytic input, directly and indirectly applied can help patients achieve some of these changes, and can contribute a lot to clinical teams' duty to provide the best risk containment possible.

Note

This is a slightly amended version of a chapter which first appeared in *Dangerous Patients: A Psychodynamic Approach to Risk Assessment and Management*, Ronald Doctor (Ed.), London: Karnac Book, 2003.

I would like to thank Dr. Leslie Sohn, my supervisor since many years, whose teaching and support is invaluable.

CHAPTER SIX

Perverse females

Their unique psychopathology

Dorothy Lloyd-Owen

The psychopathology of perversion

I shall start with some thoughts about perversion as a psychopathological entity. It is about the *absence* of a capacity to obtain sexual genital fulfilment within an intimate, loving relationship with another adult person. Instead, the individual suffering from a perversion feels taken over by compulsive behaviour (often inexplicable and bizarre to them and others) that provides temporary relief from unbearable and increasing sexualized anxiety. The notion of *temporary* relief is important, given that a feature of a perverse act is that it has to be repeated, yet it is never the hoped-for solution to intolerable psychic pain. Instead it could be thought of as an evacuation and a communication; or a repetition of early, unprocessed traumatic experiences no longer available to conscious thought.

The perverse enactment can dominate the life of the individual or be contained within a split off part of the psyche whilst the individual lives an otherwise successful and often professional life.

The source of perversion lies in a disturbed infant/mother relationship, usually with an absent father; "absent" meaning either physically not there, or physically present but uninvolved and emotionally unavailable for "containing" mother and infant or for moderating that relationship.

By disturbed infant/mother relationship, I include early or repeated indifference to the child's emotional needs, mental, physical or sexual abuse, cruelty, physical or verbal attacks and indifference to the infant's suffering. This list can also include offering the child up to paedophilic partners, cross-dressing, or subjecting the child to a psychotic parent.

A feature of the perverse individual is a longing for closeness, yet profound anxiety about engulfment and annihilation leading to hostile pulling away from the apparently desired object, usually an object that stands for the mother to the infant. Glasser described this as core complex anxiety as follows:

> In the perversions, then, the ego attempts to resolve the vicious circle of the core complex and the attendant conflicts and dangers by the widespread use of *sexualization*. Aggression is converted into sadism. The immediate consequence of this is the preservation of the mother, who is no longer threatened by total destruction, and the ensuring of the viability of the relationship to her. The intention to destroy is converted into a wish to hurt and control. Sexualization also acts as a binding, organizing force in the internal state of affairs, enabling defensive measures to be more effective and a certain stability to come about.
>
> [Glasser, 1979a, pp. 288–289]

Thus the wish to be rid of sexualized anxiety that contains unconscious hatred of the object (or, more appropriately, part object) and the perverse act, could be thought of as "making hate" rather than making love. This is most clearly seen in the paedophile who will talk of loving the child whilst doing the child physical and psychological harm.

The resultant perverse, destructive behaviour enacted in later childhood, adolescence or adulthood is an act of revenge, as if to empty the child-victim, now perpetrator, of unmanageable, still raw and unprocessed emotional pain, by pushing it into the new victim. This is a defence of identification with the aggressor, the original abandoning or attacking perpetrator (A. Freud, 1942). For many years I acted as consultant to a residential establishment that assessed abusive families. A significant number of residents came from great distances from the Centre and were often single mothers and children who had separated from an abusive man. Many found new partners in the new locality—invariably these were also abusive men. These mothers had all been abused as children and constantly recreated abusive relationships involving themselves and their children.

Clearly a physically, sexually or emotionally abused infant or child does not have the psychic, emotional or physical equipment to process abuse. We are all familiar with the knowledge that what cannot be processed emotionally has to be repeated. This is so with the abused, who—if the trauma of abuse remains unprocessed and denied by themselves and significant others—either engage others in repeating the abuse, creating an illusion of control over the victim-role, or by turning passive into active, abuse others of an age and in circumstances to mirror their own original abuse.

Shengold (1989) referred to infant and child abuse as "soul murder", something that affects and disturbs future relationships. The victim of abuse is not appreciated as a separate being, with age-appropriate capacities and feelings, but as a vehicle for whatever the abuser wants to make of him or her. An incest perpetrator or paedophile, therefore, will talk of a child as though the child had adult sexual capacities and feelings, including the capacity to seduce, desire and initiate the denied abuse.

Thus perverse functioning acts as a survival technique or organized system of defences against the earliest anxieties—for example, psychotic fragmentation, primitive confusion and disintegration, or helplessness.

Aggression and violence in the perversions

It is helpful when thinking about the function of violence and aggression in perverse acts to ask the question, as delineated by Glasser (1998), is it self-preservative or sado-masochistic? Glasser describes self-preservative violence as follows:

> We can say that aggression and violence are aroused by anything that constitutes a threat to the physical or psychological self. Thus, in a

> psychological context, this self-preservative violence is a fundamental, immediate and substantial response triggered by any threat to the self with the aim of negating this source of danger. Random illustrations of such various dangers are: attacks on one's gender identity, the danger of castration, the infliction of a blow to self-esteem, frustration, humiliation, an insult to one's self or an ideal to which one is attached, and other such external threats. Violence may also be evoked by internal events such as a loss of identity through inner confusion, feelings of disintegration, the domination by an annihilative internal object, a remorseless castigation by a tyrannical, sadistic superego, and so on. Such internal threats may be externalized so that the attack on a person may appear inexplicable. In self-mutilation or suicide, the relevant parts of the body are related to as "external" objects (see for example Campbell, 1995). Such behaviour may be regarded as a temporary psychosis but I consider it more appropriate to consider it as an extreme regression to the most primitive level of functioning and this may or may not occur in psychosis. Wolff *et al.* subscribe to such a view when they state: "The patient's underlying personality is probably an important factor in many cases of violence, even if they are mentally ill. For example, a tendency for a psychotic patient to become violent may arise from pre-morbid personality traits rather than the psychosis itself." (Wolff *et al.* 1990, p. 634)
>
> [Glasser, 1998, p. 889]

Glasser goes on, on the other hand, to describe sado-masochistic violence as follows:

> In the case of sado-masochistic violence, the response of the object is essential; the object must be seen to suffer. For example, in a war a soldier may kill one of the enemy in the interest of his survival, (self-preservative violence), while in different circumstances the soldier might kill his enemy as an act of revenge for what was done to his companions (sado-masochistic violence): or he may subject the captured enemy to bodily torture, often with great conscious pleasure (sado-masochistic violence). Thus another distinguishing feature is that an essential component of sado-masochistic violence is pleasure (which may or may not be manifest or conscious) while pleasure is not a component of self-preservative violence. The nearest self-preservative violence comes to involving pleasure is the relief when the danger is negated. (Glasser, 1998, p 891)

It is interesting to note that some women are currently pressing to be front line soldiers. It is worth thinking about what unconsciously drives this, given what we know about the unconscious motivation of non-conscripted male soldiers.

Resistance to recognizing women as perverse

In our society, perversion and especially paedophilia and incest, have male connotations, leaving women perpetrators without the help they need. The assumption is that "women do not do these things". Of course they do, but it is hard to bear the thought that mothers, our primary objects, can actively abuse or actively or unconsciously fail to protect. It is perhaps not surprising therefore that patients abused by their mothers have psychotic elements in the depth of their psychopathology. Such patients' sense of fury and grievance is often displaced onto male figures (often in a way that gives them a forensic label) with the psychological purpose of protecting the primary maternal object. It is harder to get to this by interpretations concerning the relationship with the mother, and also clinically dangerous, since collapse can be imminent when this is reached.

Perverse women can also be mis-diagnosed since, unlike their male counterparts, they perpetrate on their own bodies, or on their body products, namely their children. When they act out with others, perhaps as prostitutes or in sado-masochistic relationships, they are often regarded as having made a conscious choice, or are looked on as victims, and the solution is frequently seen as removing the male, leaving the perverse woman untreated. In the Oedipus myth the role of Jocasta is that of victim. Yet, she was more likely to have been able to recognize Oedipus as her son than he to recognize her as his mother. As in most perverse acts, the generation boundary was breached.

Since, for many, perversions are seen as the prerogative of males, this mind-set does not encompass how women act out in a perverse way. Like men, they use the reproductive system, which as a concept is more encompassing than the penis.

The main difference in male and female perversions

These were characterized by Welldon (1988) as follows:

Male perversions	*Female perversions*
1. Aimed at an "outside" object or person	1. Aimed at themselves or objects of their creation
2. Early organization around a specific perversion	2. Variable enactments of perverse psychopathology
3. No real emotional or physical attachment to the object or part object	3. Some degree of emotional or physical attachment to the object or part object
4. The action does not usually involve adult heterosexual intercourse	4. The action frequently involves adult intercourse for fantasy purposes and as a means to provide the perverse scenario
5. Desire to harm others is usually unconscious	5. Conscious desire to harm themselves. Conscious or unconscious desire to harm their babies

The core complex

Glasser refers to this constellation of anxieties as the "core complex", and writes as follows:

> When we treat perversions, we invariably come to recognize a particularly important complex of inter-related feelings, ideas, and attitudes. I refer to it as a "core complex" because the various elements that go to make it up are at the centre of the pervert's psychopathology and fundamental to it. Aggression is a major and integral element of this complex.
>
> A major component of the core complex is a deep-seated and pervasive longing for an intense and most intimate closeness to another person, amounting to a "merging", a "state of oneness", a "blissful

union". The specific versions of this longing are as varied as the individuals who express them. Such longings are, of course, by no means indicative of pathology; on the contrary, they are a component of the most normal of loving desires. However, in the pervert it persists pervasively in this most primitive form even when later developmental stages modify its manifest appearance. Such "merging" for him does not have the character of a temporary state from which he will emerge: he feels it carries with it a *permanent* loss of self, a disappearance of his existence as a separate, independent individual into the object, like being drawn into a "black hole" of space. There are individual variations depending on the particular vicissitudes of the aggressive and libidinal elements involved: of being engulfed by the object, of forcefully getting into the object or being intruded into by the object, and so on. But in one way or another the ultimate result is of being taken over totally by the object so that the anxiety is of total annihilation. This wish to merge and the consequent "annihilation anxiety" invariably comes into the transference—for example, as a fear of being "brainwashed" by the analyst, or as intensely claustrophobic feelings in the consulting room.

Among the defensive reactions provoked by this "annihilatory anxiety" is the obvious one of flight from the object, retreating emotionally to a "safe distance" (that is, essentially, a narcissistic withdrawal). This is expressed in such attitudes as placing a premium on independence and self-sufficiency. In therapy, it may be encountered as a wish to terminate treatment, as a constant argumentativeness or negativism, or the development of an intellectual detachment.

However this "flight into a safe distance" brings with it its own dangers and anxieties consequent on the implicit isolation. Such an isolated state may involve extremely painful affects and is, in my experience, one of the commonest reasons for the pervert seeking treatment. The relief from this state, or threat of it, must ultimately be sought in renewing contact with the object. Both the nature of the anxiety and the intensity of the needs cause this contact to be conceived of in terms of an indissoluble closeness, security and gratification which could only be achieved by "merging" with the object. And so there is a return to the start of the vicious circle of the core complex.

The emotional attitudes and fantasies I have described may well put one in mind of the "symbiosis" and "separation-individuation" stages of infant development (Mahler 1968) and since these stages are part of normal development it may be considered that I am not identifying anything specific to the pervert. But I would point out that the pervert differs from less severely disturbed individuals in that

> his core complex is fixated at these very early developmental stages. To envisage closeness and intimacy as annihilating, or separateness and independence as desolate isolation, indicates the persistence of a primitive level of functioning. What I have been referring to as the "object" in my description of the core complex is thus ultimately the individual's mother (or the person who functioned in that capacity) during this very early period of development (Glasser, 1979 pp. 279–280).

Case example: a female's perverse use of the body

I shall briefly describe how a young female adult perversely used her own body, both to communicate and to attempt to come to terms with her experience of being sexually abused but not penetrated by her father.

I shall not describe her complicated and initially idealized relationship with her mother whom she felt had colluded in her being abused. Nor will I describe her equally complicated relationship with her father, in which she yearned for him as a good father, whilst her rage at the way he had treated her was coloured by what we can no doubt recognize as familiar, but nonetheless inappropriate anxieties, that she had somehow colluded with him.

She was very bright, with a lot going for her, as evidenced in her being able to observe that all was not well with the way she was living her life, to link it to her earlier experience of being abused and to arrange a referral for therapy. In the referral letter her difficulties were described as follows:

> Psychosexual problems in relationships.
>
> How emotional problems were articulated through her body in:
>
> A poor relationship towards food.
> Compulsive/damaging exercising.

Perhaps we need to become accustomed to viewing such self/body relationships as the perverse enactments that they are.

What was to become the predominant transference relationship was present the first time I met her. She talked as if this was her only chance and she had to get it all out (and hopefully across to me) whilst she had my attention. During the course of the treatment, we came to understand this as me being experienced as if I were an emotionally absent, self-absorbed mother, as well as a predominantly physically absent and (when present) abusing father. My patient's experience was one of attempting to convey what it felt like to be her, but with the expectation of no real or sustained interest in her and what it felt like to be her.

The three main areas of difficulty she had described at the beginning preoccupied her throughout the treatment. We came to understand how each of them re-enacted and communicated her trauma as well as her unsuccessful attempts to master it, and her core complex anxieties which she defended against through an unconscious sado-masochistic way of relating with herself and significant others.

The difficult psychosexual relationships she referred to emerged as her having friendships that contained no sexual contact and sexual relationships that contained no friendship. These represented on the one hand her wish to have a good non-sexual relationship with a man, unconsciously representing her father, and on the other, a re-enactment of an abusive non-loving sexual contact with him. It also allowed her to turn the tables on the young men involved by breaking off sexual intercourse and telling them they reminded her of her father, which would leave them devastated, as she had been by her father's abuse. The difficulty with intimacy, which led to barren or abusive relationships, expresses core complex anxieties that, in young men, often lead to violence but in young females are frequently expressed by subtle violence against the body. She came to understand her triumph over these young men, her victims, and her own role in this as an abuser in identification with her father, as well as how her stopping something in the here and now represented her wish that she had been able to stop her abuse in the past. Also, for similar unconscious reasons she used to dress very provocatively and then repel the advances she attracted as a way of trying to process her unconscious and inappropriate self-blame.

This young woman's second preoccupation was, as she put it, emotional problems centred on her body. Whilst she recognized this she somehow managed not to see her vegetarianism moving onto veganism as an expression, for her, of emotional problems. She was, however, concerned about her compulsive exercising to the point of causing physical stress damage to herself. Again, the complexity of what this symbolized was unravelled in the treatment.

In general, both her diet and exercising were an attempt to feel an ownership of and control over her own body—what was taken in by it, and done to it, unlike her experience in relation to her father and her mother. However, both the food intake and exercise re-enacted an attack on her body. Her food intake amounted to anorexia and the exercise caused stress damage. She thus repeated, in different forms, the incestuous attack. Her non-meat eating was an unconscious attempt to control her mounting aggression towards her mother as represented by the non-consumed flesh (breast) and this was extended through veganism to anything thought of as animate.

The results of the eating pattern and exercise caused her mother considerable anxiety. In this way the young woman was able to elicit the concern she felt she had not received at the time of the abuse. It also sadistically punished her mother by causing her to feel tormented with anxiety and powerless to stop what was happening, which was how the patient felt whilst she was being abused. In many ways this young woman was more angry with her non-protective mother than with her abusing father. This has been my experience of most abused and abusing patients.

The dieting disturbed the patient's psychosexual development in as much as it stopped her periods and kept her, she thought, "child-like". This defended her against the full impact of growing up into an adult sexual woman. However, she was also concerned about this. We came to understand it as representing her anxiety that damage had been done to her "insides" by the abuse, i.e., in abusing herself she identified with her abusive father and non-protective mother. Here she felt her "insides" to be her physical body, rather than damage done to her internal world—her psyche.

From her referral, it was clear the patient understood she was seeking psychoanalytic psychotherapy. Further, there was a healthy part of her able to form a treatment alliance with me as we struggled to address the abusive her, in identification with her abuser and her non-protective mother. Central to the therapy was my need to maintain a thinking-ego/good parents' state of mind so that she could eventually mentalize rather than enact. The need to maintain a thinking stance despite intense pressure in the transference to be harsh or indifferent (abusive or non-protective) is ever present when working with patients suffering from perversions. In this case, it needed thoughtful care not to be drawn into superego-ish comments when I was the container of her anxieties about the damage she was doing to herself, not to re-enact in the therapy room the maternal object who asserted "it's *your fault*". Equal care to think and not to act–re-enact was essential in not defending against these anxieties by being experienced, like her father, as indifferent to her suffering.

The therapy had the outcome of her giving up her symptoms. She ceased the compulsive exercises, improved her diet so that her menstrual cycle resumed, and she formed a more loving sexual relationship. However, like many young women, she left treatment "to get on with her life" when her symptoms had abated, whilst in part knowing further therapy was needed. Some years after treatment ended she wrote a moving letter in which it was clear that the work still to be done was recognized by her, but was able to be experienced as psychic pain, rather than enacted as self-abuse, or abuse of those to whom she was attached.

Transference and counter-transference and issues of technique

The perverse patient has a particular relationship to her superego that is not experienced as benign. Instead it can be cruelly abusive, attacking or corrupt. The relationship to such a superego demands compliance or is dealt with by defiance—there is no hope of the to and fro of dialogue, since it is made up of narcissistic, or abusive, or absent and therefore non-protective internalizations. The perverse female has in childhood become the container, rather than the contained. Such patients might be designated as borderline. Rosenfeld (1978) puts this succinctly, albeit referring to males, as follows:

> The borderline patient who is dominated by confusional anxieties and pathological splitting processes has to be clearly distinguished from *the destructive narcissistic patient*, as he is unable to face interpretations of a destructive self even if it is clearly exposed in dreams. Detailed examination reveals that he is in the grip of a primitive superego structure where positive, often highly erotic and seductive features are mixed up with omnipotent, sadistically overpowering ones. The demands of this superego are very contradictory and

> therefore confusing and impossible for the patient to cope with, as it creates at first some doubt, but ultimately complete uncertainty and confusion in the patient. When this primitive superego is projected on to the analyst and he interprets destructive aspects in the patient that are clearly shown in the material, in dreams and in projection into other people, the patient is overwhelmed with anxiety because he hears the analyst saying that he is 100 per cent bad. This threatens his whole self with death, disintegration and madness, for he will try to find omnipotent ways of escaping from this danger. The patient in this state is unable to think about his own problems and impulses because he has lost the capacity for self-observation, and all his attention is focused on the analyst who, in the patient's perception, sees the patient as extremely bad and destructive. To defend himself against this catastrophe the patient becomes icily defensive; in addition, he identifies himself with the primitive superego and accuses the analyst in a very violent manner. The patient is severely shocked in this situation because interpretations have a terrifying effect on him; he feels that the analyst, like his mother, had not been able to introject and understand the patient's projected primitive superego. At that moment the process of projective identification gets out of hand and a transference psychosis becomes manifest where the patient misperceives the analyst and sees him as his superego.
>
> [Rosenfeld, 1978, p. 217]

Therapists may need a supervisor's help in framing interventions in a way that is as free as possible from being perceived as abusive and humiliating. However, since this is inevitable, consideration of how to take up the patient's feeling when this happens is crucial. For the perverse patient, the very fact of being in therapy, of coming to a session, can feel terrifying since the transference is to an abusive or non-protecting object. For example, I recall a patient who, regarding herself as trans-sexual, engaged in sadistic attacks on myself and the therapy by threatening to go to Charing Cross Hospital "to have the operation" and on one occasion graphically described to me what would happen to me if I went and had the operation. Thus I, not her, was subjected to this cruel and mutilating process. It was then essential to be able to think about both process and content rather than get caught up in it by feeling exasperated and at the patient's mercy, or sadistically retaliating, thereby enacting her violent superego. At times a supervisor's capacity to think about how the therapist can be pulled into enactment and what this is defending against is vital since it triangulates the interaction.

Such patients will, by projection, pull you into being superego or id if at all possible, when what is needed is good ego functioning. In the experience of most perverse patients there has been an absence of triangulation in their early histories. Parents have not been available as a thinking (ego) couple but instead there has been the experience of a cruel, superego figure and an id—"anything goes" figure. It needs to be remembered that to the child, the parent who does not know abuse is being perpetrated is experienced as giving permission for the abuse to take place.

The sado-masochistic compliant/defiant transference is very subtle. We may offer an interpretation or insight and feel it is welcome and used, only to discover it is used as a defensive compliance to avoid *real* contact, a *real* relationship which for most perverse patients is a profoundly dangerous experience, against which a great deal of their overt and covert acting out defends. The force of the attack on thinking and the pull towards superego or id responses are powerful in the transferences. Putting it another way, the pull towards acting out (as for example the patient provokes the therapist in the counter-transference to act as the abuser, or non-protector) is ever present at the expense of thinking and containing.

I recall a patient organized around a sado-masochistic lifestyle that involved frequenting S&M clubs and parties as well as being known for being available for one-plus-one S&M sessions in the higher echelons of society. She also led an otherwise self-abusive lifestyle including massive debts. She evacuated her anxiety about these into me. In one session she related how her debts were about to be cleared by a highly lucrative S&M engagement. I recall my powerful experience of relief in the counter-transference (id/non-protective) and it took time to recover my capacity to think and not then to react in an abusive superego way.

Thus deception and corruption, attacks and non-protectiveness are ever present in the process and content of therapeutic work with perverse patients. It is imperative to hold on to the knowledge that they are both victims and perpetrators. The perpetration can be on objects or internal objects, parts of self attacking and abusing other parts of self. Invariably, it is a cruel part of self in identification with the abuser or non-protector, attacking and denigrating a healthy, needy, vulnerable, appropriately dependent and seeking a dependable object, part of self.

It is important to take the patient's anxiety about abuse in the consulting room seriously. This is often present and can be interpreted as the patient's fear of what she may do to you or you may do to her. I recall seeing a patient for a first assessment session. Once in my room she looked at me from a white-mask face that terrified me and it took me time to realize it was her terror I was experiencing. I put this into words and she was able to say she was terrified of what I would say. This is a patient who for many years remained in bed apart from once weekly shopping and once weekly attendance for her sessions. In bed she felt safe and protected from her perverse acting out and fear of attacks from others onto whom she projected her violence. She had been abandoned by her mother at age 2 and left in the care of her violent father. Subsequently, she was abused sexually by a neighbour. She has a criminal history.

Workers may defend against their anxiety by becoming oblivious to the danger or be so anxious that they cannot name what is happening. It helps to be able to say something that takes up both sides of the patient's dilemma, such as, "You want me to be anxious, otherwise I would not know how serious it is, but not so anxious that I cannot be of use to you?" Thus one hopes to re-establish oneself as a container, as ego rather than superego or id, as previously stated, or as parents who can think together, instead of one abusing and one not knowing. This is a different experience from that of the parents of the patients I have described. It often needs a supervisor to name this process.

It is important, when working with such clients, to be in a containing setting and to provide a containing setting—this applies not only to the consulting room and state of mind of the worker, but also demands clarity about confidentiality before treatment starts. If working in an agency or institution it is important to be clear with the patient about the agency's policy of violating confidentiality. At the Portman Clinic, where the patients have so far been assured of confidentiality, we arrange where necessary for a colleague to act as case manager and to respond to the concerns coming from the outside world.

Conclusion

Firstly, I cannot over-emphasize the importance of thought over action in the face of the pressure for action such patients exert on both individuals and institutions. For the therapist, the struggle to maintain a thinking space and a capacity to think is critical in the face of activity as defence. This facilitates the patient's development of a capacity to mentalize.

Secondly, I consider the triangulation of supervision very important when working with such patients who have rarely experienced a good containing couple with consequent difficulties around Oedipal resolution.

Thirdly, I want to emphasize the importance of information gathering and history taking, given the early, indeed pre-verbal trauma and its legacy in such patients. This goes in and out of fashion in psychoanalysis but is essential in the roots of a perverse defence.

Fourthly, the therapist needs containment, hopefully provided by the agency setting to allow work with this difficult patient group.

Finally, perverse women do not in the main turn to outsiders to try to master or communicate their own earlier abuse. They use the whole of their own bodies and their babies for this purpose. What goes into or comes out of their bodies is used to express not love but hate or revenge. What should be creative becomes perverse—the death instinct predominates over the life instinct, bad objects are idealized and good objects denigrated. The aim of the behaviour is to destroy any knowledge of need, dependency and vulnerability again, just as it had been when the original abuse occurred. Thus the penis is denigrated in acts of prostitution or sado-masochism, babies and children are abused or unconsciously offered up to others for abuse, food is not used as nourishment but in the service of bulimia and anorexia, and the skin is not experienced as a containing boundary of self but as something to be attacked and penetrated by cuts and the insertion of (usually) sharp metal objects. It is therefore important that the perverse psychopathology is recognized as such and treated in a way that gives due weight both to the victim and the perpetrator within the patient.

Note

This chapter was previously published in *British Journal of Psychotherapy, 19*(3) 2003 pp. 285–296.

CHAPTER SEVEN

From biting teeth to biting wit

The normative development of aggression[1]

Marianne Parsons

> [A] little girl of three, in the throes of a struggle with her rather wild aggressive nature . . . returned one day from nursery school to report triumphantly on her "good" behaviour in the group: "Not hit, not kick, not bit, only spit!"
>
> [A. Freud, 1972, p. 163]

The concept of aggression is one of the most controversial in psychoanalytic theory. Views range from seeing aggression as an instinctual drive on a par with libido, the derivation of the death instinct, an expression of the self-preservative instincts, a reaction to environmental influences. It can be understood in terms of activity, adaptation and mastery, and as destructive and pathological. The theoretical viewpoint we take profoundly affects our clinical understanding and technique.

The capacity for aggression is essential for psychic growth. The healthy development of the self and the capacity to separate and individuate require aggressive activity. Like sexuality, aggression can be used constructively and progressively, or destructively and regressively. Its appropriateness in any specific situation depends on the manner of its expression and the developmental level of the individual. For example, it is age appropriate for a toddler to have tantrums, but not the older child or adolescent. In situations of real danger, violent aggression to protect the self or others may be entirely appropriate. On the other hand, such behaviours as unprovoked violence, sadism, contemptuous denigration, bullying and wanton destructiveness are largely regressive and arise from pathology, not health. Because of their regressive and pathological nature there is no developmental line for such destructive behaviours. By contrast, one can conceive of a developmental line of normative healthy aggression and an attempt will be made in this paper to trace this, together with some of the influences that can throw it off course.

Winnicott's view was that aggression arises from environmental impingements, especially traumatic early object experiences, as well as instinctual forces (Winnicott, 1950–1955). Summarizing a panel on aggression, Heimann and Valenstein wrote:

> Our psychoanalytic experience tells us that certain patients who show particular problems with aggression have had to suppress or otherwise defend themselves in infancy and childhood from environmental influences that were not conducive to the progression of their developmental needs for the normal expression of aggression.
>
> [Heimann and Valenstein, 1972, p. 34]

The power of love to bind hatred is crucial. People showing pathological aggression tend to be those who were not enabled in childhood to develop a secure libidinal attachment in which they felt loved and contained by primary caretakers. Institutionalized children with multiple caretakers, traumatized children and those who have suffered severe physical pain, neglect or over-stimulation, and children for whom fear has been a daily currency may show the kind of uncontrollable, apparently senseless destructiveness otherwise only seen in brain-damaged and psychotic children. Anna Freud noted that the pathological factor in such cases was not the aggressive tendencies themselves, but a lack of fusion between the aggressive and libidinal urges:

> The pathological factor is found in the realm of erotic, emotional development that has been held up through adverse external or

> internal conditions, such as absence of love objects, lack of emotional response from the adult environment, breaking of emotional ties as soon as they are formed, deficiency of emotional development for innate reasons. Owing to the defects on the emotional side, the aggressive urges are not brought into fusion and thereby bound and partially neutralised, but remain free and seek expression in life in the form of pure, unadulterated, independent destructiveness . . . The appropriate therapy has to be directed to the neglected, defective side, i.e. the emotional libidinal development.
>
> [A. Freud, 1949, pp. 41–42]

There is a danger of equating adult behaviours, feelings and fantasies with those of children. Something may look actively destructive to our adult eye, but we should not assume that destructive intent (as we know it) is necessarily in the young child's mind. The child's capacity for mental functioning is limited at every developmental stage by his awareness of himself and his knowledge of the world around him. Does the tiny baby who screams and kicks have destructive intent, or is he in some primitive bodily way trying to get rid of intolerable feelings? Edgcumbe (1976) addressed this question succinctly:

> The baby's wish to get rid of nasty experiences may be viewed as the earliest form of mental aggressiveness in the sense that it involves a primitive hostile reaction to something unpleasant. The very young baby, however, cannot tell what the something is, where it comes from, or what, if wishing does not work, will make it go away. He cannot distinguish between feelings arising in his own body and stimuli coming from outside.
>
> [Edgcumbe, 1976, p. vii]

The baby gradually begins to differentiate 'me' from 'not-me' and inner experience from external stimuli, learning over time that his cries prompt his mother to do something to relieve his distress. When his cries go unheard and his needs unmet, he begins to feel frustrated. The baby needs "perfect adaptation at the theoretical start, and then needs a carefully graduated failure of adaptation" (Winnicott, 1950–1955, p. 216). Crucial for the development of the sense of a real self and the capacity for healthy relationships is the opposition the mother offers to the young child, the importance of the child's experience of aggression and the need for fusion between erotic love and aggression (Winnicott, 1950–1955). Aggression therefore operates both in the service of self-preservation and survival *and* development.

The development of aggression is closely connected with many aspects of the child's development: psychosexual, object relations, ego and superego, cognitive capacities and the integration of his sense of self. All these contribute to the child's abilities (or not) to tolerate, process, and deal with his aggressive feelings at every stage of development. There are developmentally appropriate fantasies and means of expressing, defending against and dealing with aggression—hence the title of this paper, which implies a movement from bodily to symbolic expression.

Infancy—"From biting teeth . . ."

In the oral phase of infancy, feeling hungry, feeling full, swallowing, biting, spitting, vomiting, gurgling, cooing and crying play a key role in the experience and expression of pleasure and unpleasure (S. Freud, 1920). Privation or frustration of basic needs and of a sense of going-on-being (Winnicott, 1963a) can arouse primitive anxieties of disintegration and annihilation. Observation indicates that the earliest forms of aggression are triggered by such primitive *anxieties*, not by wilful innate destructiveness.

The adult's loving expression "I could eat you!" aptly mirrors the aggressive possessive love that the baby has for his mother (stemming originally, we imagine, from his attitude towards her feeding breast). This aggressive possessive love can be seen in the way children love their most beloved toys "to death", biting off their ears, flinging them aside, then retrieving and clutching them passionately. At this stage of development it is *aggressive love* not *hatred* that threatens destruction (A. Freud, 1949). The baby's intimacy with the mother is conducted primarily through bodily expressions. Typical signs of protest are gaze avoidance, refusing food and squirming when being held. Self-directed aggression (biting, head-banging and hair-pulling) is unusual and indicates disturbance (Hoffer, 1949).

> From this stage of development onwards it is essential for the child's normality that the aggressive urges should be directed away from the child's own body to the animate or inanimate objects in the environment . . . At a later stage aggression will normally be used again in a self-destructive manner. But it will then be invested in the superego and directed against the ego itself, not against the body.
>
> [A. Freud, 1949, p. 40]

Although babies may be endowed with differing strengths of aggressive drive, the impact of the environment on the child's capacity to deal with aggressive forces is crucial. How babies begin to make sense of their feelings and experiences depends largely on the way the mother perceives and relates to them, which will be affected by her own internal world and experiences of self and other. The mother's capacity to empathize with and help her baby manage his greedy demands will be impaired if she feels too plagued by his cries, experiencing them as attacks. This will impede the baby's healthy aggressive development.

> When a tiny baby feels hungry or frightened he has no resources for making himself feel better and has to rely on his caregivers. If his needs are not adequately met, his distress, helplessness and sense of frustration will become overwhelming. He will yell and cry, kick and flail his arms. This constitutes the earliest mode of response to an overwhelming experience, namely a bodily one. The crucial thing from the point of view of development is the nature of the mother's response. Good-enough mothering will give the baby sufficiently often an experience of not yelling and flailing into a vacuum, but of having elicited a response that alleviates his distress. This is more than the meeting of a need; it is the meeting up with an empathic and receptive object. It lays the foundations for the capacity to tolerate vulnerability because helplessness is associated with a protective object.
>
> [Parsons & Dermen, 1999, pp. 330–331]

The good-enough mother acts as a protective shield (S. Freud, 1920; Khan, 1973) by empathic attunement to her baby and by trying to relieve her baby's pain and anxiety until he gradually develops the resources to do this for himself. This enables the baby to develop a sense of basic safety and trust, to have pleasurable experiences with the mother and to form a secure attachment to her. Not only does the baby feel loved, but he also develops over time a capacity to attune to his own internal states, tolerate his needs and differentiate between shades of feeling until not every internal state has the same urgency. Prolonged absence of the mother's protective function exposes the baby to unmanageable amounts of anxiety that can lead to a deviant course of aggression and patterns of relating (Fraiberg, 1982). A mother's protective function may be inadequate for many reasons, for example, depression, unresolved conflicts over her own aggression, unconscious hostility to her baby, lack of support from her partner.

As the baby begins to develop a sense of self-agency (Stern, 1985), the good-enough mother intuitively recognizes that her baby can tolerate more frustration and can exercise his curiosity and do more things for himself. She continues to "feel with" her baby (Furman, 1992) but, instead of immediately managing her baby's feelings for him, she gives him more space to begin to learn how to manage his own feelings and experiences. The baby begins to internalize her protective function. Repeated experiences of optimal frustration in the context of empathic mothering help him learn that he can survive feelings of helplessness without being overwhelmed. This promotes the development of healthy aggression.

A vignette from mother–infant observation illustrates a baby's aggressive reaction to anxiety, fear and distress within a good-enough mother–child relationship.

> K is 10 months old. Her mother went away for three days and she slept a lot during this time. When the mother returned K did not look at her, only at the window, and when the mother went to the car to collect her luggage, K cried and cried in absolute despair as if it was all too much for her to bear. For the next three days K guarded the door, but then was able to settle and feel safe again. When I visited one week later, K came to greet me with her shoe in her hand. We had played a very nice game with her shoe on previous visits—she would give it to me, and I would give it back. At first I thought she wanted to play the game again, but this time she came closer to me, holding the shoe in the air. I thought she was going to hit me so I made a move to defend myself, but she just stopped in front of me holding the shoe high in the air. She looked at me seriously, then turned round, crawled over to the wall and began to hit the wall with the shoe. Her

> mother said, "No, K, that will mark the wall." K listened to her and stopped hitting the wall, then went over to her toys. She began to throw her toys in the air, listening to the hard noise they made as they fell to the floor. The mother seemed to understand K's state of mind and said, "Good girl!".
>
> [R. Pohjamo, personal communication, 1994]

K's aggressiveness seems to stem from her reaction to mother's absence. Although not physically aggressive towards her mother, she had clearly been distressed (she could not look at mother when she returned, cried in absolute despair, then guarded the door for 3 days). When the observer arrives—someone who regularly comes and goes—we can imagine K remembering her feelings about mother's absence and return, and surmise that K's aggression towards mother is displaced in her aggressive approach to the observer. But instead of attacking she displaces her aggression onto the wall. When mother prohibits this, she displaces her aggressive feelings further into a game, throwing her toys and enjoying the hard noise they make. The observer senses that mother knows that K is displacing her aggressive feelings onto inanimate objects as she encourages this adaptive behaviour by praising her for being a "good girl". Perhaps K's secure relationship with her mother enables her to remember her love for mother and wish to please her even in the face of aggressive feelings towards her, i.e. the foundations of the fusion between libidinal and aggressive urges.

Toddlers

The toddler continues to express aggression via the body (biting, kicking, pinching, throwing things) and through screams and yells because he has not yet developed the mental resources for processing and managing feelings of frustration and anger. Prior to developing the capacity for concern for the object, the toddler revels in a sense of powerful agency and some cruelty is to be expected at this age (Winnicott, 1963b). Cruelty to animals is not uncommon: the family pet often needs to be rescued both from the toddler's attacks and his aggressive love. Toddlers feel omnipotent, resent being controlled or having to share. They delight in being messy, noisy, powerful and aggressive. Aggression is triggered especially by assaults on the child's omnipotence, by fear of loss of the object and of the object's love, and by core complex anxieties of feeling abandoned or engulfed (Glasser, 1996). Advances in ego development allow for a wider variety of defences. For example, when the toddler's messy or cruel wishes conflict with his internal and/or external world, he may deal with them by attempting to transform them into the opposite through 'reaction formation'. Thus cruelty may be transformed into pity, kindness and protectiveness. Reaction formation is a very adaptive, civilizing defence; but if over-used or used precociously, it can lead to maladaptive ways of defending against aggressive impulses such as pathological self-sacrifice, perfectionism and obsessionality.

At this stage, magical thinking holds sway: to wish something makes it happen. There is no clear distinction between reality and fantasy or between internal and external events. So, the angry toddler who is left by his mother may imagine that his wish to get rid of her made her disappear. It takes time to sort this out. It also takes time for the toddler to learn that the adults perceive some things they do whilst exploring their environment as dangerous, destructive or naughty. The toddler faces the confusing problem:

> which of his many activities are really destructive or aggressive, and which are potentially useful and creative? In normal development the child gradually arrives at some kind of working definition that allows him to distinguish between those of his actions that are actually harmful and those which are not.
>
> [Edgcumbe, 1976, p. x]

During healthy toddler-hood the child begins to assert more independence by actively doing more for himself, in *his* way. But the toddler also wants to please mother because his well-being depends on her love. He faces a major conflict of ambivalence as he experiences violent swings between love and hate. He hates mum when she does not gratify him but loves her when she comforts and provides for his needs. When the toddler feels hatred, his sense of loving and being loved may disappear. Such intense feelings arise in relation to many age-appropriate developmental conflicts. Toilet training is an obvious example where faeces (a loving gift or a noxious weapon) may be used as an expression of love or aggression in the mother–child relationship. (Derivatives of this type of anal aggressiveness sometimes persist into later life as expressions of contempt. In extreme forms they appear in some types of criminality, e.g. the burglar who literally leaves shit everywhere.) If the mother can manage her toddler's anger and hatred without feeling narcissistically wounded, without retaliating and without needing to deny his negative feelings towards her, she offers him a model for dealing with ambivalence. Through internalization of her capacities, the child integrates his loving views of the mother with the angry and hostile ones, and recognizes that the mum who is sometimes angry with him also still loves him. This integration of loving and hating feelings is crucial for the healthy development of aggression. It enables the child to develop a sense of trust that his affectionate relationship with mother will endure during moments of anger and separations from her. Without such integration, "omnipotent and magical ways of thinking will persist unmodified, the power of love to tame destructiveness will be diminished, and the child's belief in the enormity of his aggression will be unchecked" (Parsons & Dermen, 1999, p. 333).

Increasingly, the mother has to say "no" to stop the toddler in order to protect him from danger, or to protect herself and others from his aggressive behaviour. He *must not* bite his sister or make a mess, he *should* use the potty, put on his coat, etc. Such limits and demands make him feel frustrated and angry, forcing him to recognize that he is not all-powerful and will not be gratified unconditionally. This painful blow to his previously omnipotent sense of himself arouses enormous frustration and often results in the temper tantrums typical in toddler-hood. The toddler in a tantrum can feel overwhelmed and out of control, and needs the continuous presence of the adult to help him regain composure. Being angrily controlled or left alone in such a state leaves the child at the mercy of unmanageable panic and does not help him to learn ways of containing and dealing with his frustration and aggression. The parents' ability to treat the child with respect and enable him to feel a 'somebody' (Furman, 1992) while imposing restraints offers the child a model for internalization, whereby he can develop an active sense of self and self-respect and an acceptance of limits.

Observations from a Mother–Toddler Group illustrate the

development of aggression at this stage. Mrs. A, a loving and attentive mother, was anxious to avoid any confrontation with Tom. Nervous of any signs of aggression, she was never firm with him, but she was very controlling in her attempts to help him. Tom was very tied to her and wanted to be babied. He could not assert himself and found no delight in age-appropriate aggressive play or behaviour.

> Just before he was two, Tom made a tower of blocks. His mother intervened to show him how to place them correctly. He built as directed, then pushed over the tower without any delight. Very cautiously he began to build again, but doing it his way with the blocks in a haphazard fashion.
>
> Two weeks later, Tom had found a little more self-assertiveness. Tom put the little Russian dolls together in the wrong order, and his mum repeatedly showed him the correct way, explaining carefully all the time. Finally, Tom covered the doll's face with another piece, and shouted triumphantly, "Can't talk!"

Good for Tom! His first moves towards self-assertion and individuation were a struggle, but gradually he became more independent and assertive. His fantasy play provided an imaginative outlet for the expression of his aggressive urges, his need to feel in control, and his burgeoning thoughts about being a phallic boy. When Tom's father began to spend more time with him, their deeper relationship facilitated Tom's capacity to individuate from the intense and rather intrusive relationship with mother. He began to develop a stronger masculine identification and his fantasy play took on a more aggressive and phallic quality, with age-appropriate games and stories about guns and swords.

The parents' capacity to tolerate and manage their own frustration and aggression allows them to perceive their child's aggression as that of a child and enables them to respond appropriately as an adult instead of reacting on the basis of their own childlike needs and impulses. They offer experiences of forgiveness and reparation that promote the development of a healthy and non-punitive superego, and the way in which they defend against their own aggression will be internalized by the child. The child has repeated opportunities to see that aggression may be felt but not acted on, expressed in an assertive but not damaging way or channelled into other activities.

He learns that language is usually more appropriate than bodily expressions of aggression. All this promotes the child's natural urge to master feelings, conflicts and anxieties that, in turn, enhances his self-esteem and sense of well-being.

The nursery-school child

At this age the child is particularly preoccupied with curiosity about sexual differences and wishes to be big, strong and admired. In boys this centres especially on physical and phallic power; in girls it is more about power to possess and exclude others. Aggression may be triggered by anxiety over loss of love, jealousy, envy and castration anxiety, and especially by affronts to the child's narcissism (causing him to feel shamefully small, humiliated, and like a dependent baby). Interestingly, the majority of violent adult men seen at the Portman Clinic, have severe problems with phallic narcissism.

Strides in ego development offer an increasing array of defences for dealing with unwelcome wishes, impulses and fantasies. One of the most common is externalization, which 'gives the problem' to someone or something else—the childhood version of "not me, guv!"—whereby the child can feel virtuous by identifying someone else as the naughty, aggressive or guilty one. However, the problem can easily ricochet back onto the child when externalization extends to projection: the child then fears attack from the one he imbued with aggression. This is the source of many typical childhood fears of ghosts, monsters, wild animals and burglars. If defences for dealing with aggressive urges break down and aggressive wishes threaten to become conscious, nightmares may ensue and anything that might trigger conflictual feelings (such as stories, TV programmes, fantasy play, competitive and physical games) may become a source of fear to be avoided. The child may become phobic and inhibited. Aggression may be turned against the self and the child may become accident-prone.

Some aggression is essential for separation. If the child's ego cannot tolerate aggressive feelings because they seem too dangerous, he may be unable to separate. For example, the child may fear leaving mum to start school because of his unconscious death wishes towards her, so he has to stay by her side to ensure that she remains safe. This is at the root of much school refusal and school phobia in childhood and adolescence.

I have been referring to defences that may be adaptive in the service of development or maladaptive impeding development. What of children without defences against aggression? At the mercy of their impulses, all hell will break loose: not only do they damage people and things, they also damage relationships and the chance of having experiences that help them to feel good about themselves. Material about Charles illustrates this.

> Charles, aged 6, was referred for analysis because of eruptive aggression, an inability to relate to peers and alarming swings between infantile behaviour and pseudo-mature language. He was terrified of abandonment, perceiving himself as a "devil" hated by his parents. He was sure I would hate him too. His physical attacks on me were very violent: sometimes he behaved like a wild animal, spitting, biting, kicking, hurling toys, smearing faeces. His apparently unprovoked and unpredictable attacks were not simply manifestations of rage, but enactments of his internal chaos driven by panic. In time I understood that he was experiencing me, in the transference, as the source of danger. He enacted his internal chaos because he lacked resources for processing his emotional experiences in symbolic form, either through play or words, and he had no effective defences in the face of overwhelming internal states. Interpretation only heightened his anxiety and hence his aggression, instead of offering relief. By surviving without retaliating, by trying to offer a sense of safety and containment and by trying to let him know that I wanted to help, not harm, him, it gradually became possible to find a therapy 'language' that made words meaningful yet safe. When he was relatively calm and not actually 'spilling' out his chaos, I tried to empathize with his need for "body talk" to express his "spilly feelings". My aim was both to keep him safe and enable him to begin to internalize a protective function. The first step was to help him to recognize an impending danger (approach of "spilly feelings"), which would allow him to prepare himself by using anxiety as a signal (S. Freud, 1926). The next step was to help him find some appropriate defences to deal with his anxiety. Gradually he began to express and explore his terrifying fantasies in play rather than violent "body talk". The gradual development of signal anxiety, together with his emerging capacities for some symbolic play, for differentiating reality

> from fantasy and for using words meaningfully, provided him with resources for developing appropriate defences to deal with his anxiety and aggression.

Charles was a very disturbed child who seemed to have had the worst of both worlds: an intensely powerful aggressive drive coupled with an uncontaining and often hostile environment. He felt hated by his parents and his mother's unconscious death wishes towards him were palpable. His emotional development was severely delayed and lacking the phallic-narcissistic and Oedipal characteristics typical for a child of his age (Edgcumbe & Burgner, 1975).

Normally, nursery-school aged children are passionately curious about their own and others' genitals, and they puzzle about their functions. The mental images aroused by this confusion may lead them to imagine sexual activity as fighting. The child's longings for admiration, together with his passionate and aggressive interest in sexual activity, come to a head at the Oedipal level in a conflict between his active wish to possess one parent exclusively and his anxiety about damaging his rival, the other parent. He wants to get rid of the rival, but fears retaliation for his aggressive wishes. He also faces the thorny problem that his rival is someone he still loves and needs. In a good-enough family environment, children find some resolutions of this dilemma by using their increasing capacities for rational thinking, reality testing, frustration tolerance and delayed gratification. Further ego development promotes capacities for symbolization and distinguishing between reality and fantasy, allowing aggressive urges to be channelled through fantasy and play.

Physical expressions of aggression are still common at this stage, but the healthy child will increasingly use language to hurl insults. Repetitive chanting such as "Silly you! Silly poo!" is typical. Although some cruelty to animals is expectable in toddler-hood, such cruelty in the nursery-aged child is usually a sign that the fusion of aggression with love and concern has stalled, causing the normative development of aggression to veer off course.

Latency

Physical aggression tends to be more purposeful and within fairly well defined limits, unlike the rather random quality typical in younger children. Playground fights involving both physical and verbal aggression are quite commonplace in latency. If cruelty to animals persists into latency, serious disturbance is indicated. Persistent physical aggression is now a cause for concern.

In early latency, when the superego is not yet fully internalized, children believe firmly that others should be fair to them, but that they need not be fair to others. Aggression in competitive games takes the form of guiltless cheating, until the superego becomes more consolidated and the importance of fairness all round takes root. The child begins to adhere to the unwritten code that it is wrong to attack someone smaller or weaker; to take what is not yours and one against many is unfair. Children without the kind of internal world and good-enough home environment that promotes this kind of fair-minded thinking and capacity to restrain aggressive impulses, may show signs of delinquency and unrestrained aggression, and may become bullies.

With some resolution of Oedipal conflicts and solid foundations for gender identity, the development of the healthy latency child moves apace. His sense of self as capable of *doing* things and of *being* someone progresses alongside the development of the ego ideal. Progressive ego and superego capacities provide the child with a broader variety of defences and offer more adaptive means of mastering and channelling his impulses and processing feelings. Language plays a central role in the expression of aggression and the child channels his energies into fantasy, constructive play and learning. Competitiveness is directed into sports and typical latency activities, such as collecting things. The passionate hunger for information and activities reveals the sublimation of instinctual urges. Developing the capacity for sublimation is a remarkable achievement and opens up new horizons for self-enhancing interests and activities, often giving pleasure not only to the child but to others too. However, development does not proceed this smoothly for some children whose progress is impeded by their defences.

Ben, aged 7, was referred for treatment because his parents were worried about his wish to dress up as a girl in fantasy games. He was anxious about separating from his mum, jealous of his older sister and his little brother and, although usually very quiet, he would sometimes explode in rage. His wish to act the baby at home irritated his mother enormously. For many weeks in therapy he arranged the toy cars or animals in a long line, then moved the first car forward an inch followed by each car next in line. He then repeated the whole painstaking process again and again. It was painful and deadly boring to watch, and terribly sad to see his tremendous anxiety about his sexual and aggressive impulses reflected in his inhibited and strictly controlled play. Gradually he showed me more of himself but he remained frightened and ashamed of his feelings and thoughts, and anxious that I would be disapproving or intrusive like his mum, so he often needed to shut me out.

Walking downstairs at the end of a silent session, he said, "It's very dark and I'm going to die." The next day he was reluctant to come to the room and then silently read a comic. After a while I said, "I remember what you said yesterday. It was very important. You were really scared and couldn't tell me anything until you were leaving. Do you remember?" He said no. I tried again, "I remember that you said it was very dark and you were going to die. It was such a scary feeling that you hardly dared to tell me. But you did, and that was very brave . . ." He said he didn't want to talk about it, but a bit later he said, "When I'm in bed at night I worry about a war, about a bomb coming through the roof ... But I don't want to talk about it." I reminded him that a few weeks ago he hadn't wanted to talk about his worry about going to the dentist, but he had been able to be brave enough to tell me and the talking had helped. "Mm," he said. "It wasn't a worry about having my teeth pulled out." We remembered that he'd been terrified that he would not wake up from the anaesthetic. "Yes ... I'm going to forget about it ... But I can't ... I keep dreaming about it. I dream that I'm a doctor doing that to someone else. It's better to do it to someone than have it done to you." I said, "Yes, imagining scaring and hurting someone else is a way of trying to manage the worry."

The following day we played draughts. I said the game was a bit like a battle with two armies fighting. When he moved his white pieces, he used a baby voice to make the piece talk about moving forward but staying safe. Soon it became clear that he was playing out a fantasy in which the babies (his white pieces) were going to be killed by the grown-ups (my black pieces). In order to stay alive, the

> babies had to kill the murderous parents, but the babies were captured, put in prison and had their heads chopped off. As each baby was beheaded, it joined with another "dead" baby until he ended up with one enormous white piece made up of all the previously "dead" pieces. As the white piece increased in size, it became the "king", then the "queen", "King Kong", the "bla-bla monster", the "double bla-bla monster", and finally the "triple bla-bla monster". It was all-powerful and stronger than all my black "adult" pieces. I said, "So, the biggest baby triple bla-bla monster in the whole world feels safe at last because no-one can capture or kill him and he is powerful enough to kill all the parents." Ben grinned with triumph. At the end of the session he carefully put the counters in the box in pairs, but surprisingly with a black and a white one in each pair. I asked, "Do some of the babies want to be back with their parents?" In a baby voice, he replied, "Yes, but some don't." I talked about the baby part of Ben feeling so scared and cross with his parents that he wanted to kill them—but that was such a scary thought that he imagined instead that *they* were murderers, but that was terrifying too. I said that all the killing feelings felt just too awful and he preferred to forget them all. "Yes . . . like the bomb worry . . . it's the baby bit of me that gets very scared, and the big part tells the baby part it's safe and there are no wars and no bombs."

Ben felt utterly overwhelmed by his aggressive impulses and anger towards his parents, especially mother, and consequently was afraid of separating from her. His massive defences against aggression severely restricted his life. Eventually we discovered his fantasy that if he could be a girl or a baby he would be free of the turmoil of his anxiety and destructive aggression. Analysis of his fears, fantasies and defences (especially concerning aggression) enabled him to want to grow up into a man and freed him to enter a more typical and enjoyable latency.

Puberty and adolescence

At puberty children are besieged by increasing sexual and aggressive forces as their bodies undergo massive physical and hormonal changes, giving rise to much anxiety and confusion. As their bodies mature, they face the excitement, responsibilities, fantasies and fears that accompany the approach of adulthood, including the reality that they will soon be as big, powerful and sexually active as the parents. This feels potentially exciting *and* lonely and terrifying. Pubertal children experience an enormous sense of loss of their childhood body image and of mother as their chief caretaker (Laufer, 1981). Previously, they could rely on adults intervening if their aggression got out of hand, but their increased physical strength means taking further responsibility for the damage their body could do.

Adolescents typically struggle with the conflict of wishing to be looked after like a dependent child (regressive wishes which they also defend against) and wanting to become an independent adult (which they also fear). Alongside this, they struggle to find an identity that will make them feel good about themselves. To defend against fears of regression, dependence and passivity, they may develop a self-image of being invulnerable, independent and aggressive. Although this is more obvious in adolescent boys, for whom conflicts of passivity and dependence arouse age-typical homosexual anxieties, the following shows some of the roots of this conflict in an adolescent girl:

> At 18, Lisa had a breakdown at University. Her sado-masochistic style of relating had caused her to lose friends and boyfriends, but she apparently revelled in the image of herself as a "tough, provocative bitch". She was attempting to defend against conflicts over regression and dependence, and trying to find some kind of stable self-image in defiance of a sadistic superego that impatiently demanded perfection. Such a harsh superego undermined any good feelings about herself and she resorted to rebelling and giving free rein to her destructiveness as temporary means to raise her self-esteem. She said, "If I feel depressed, I have to fight. It's the only way I know of relating to people and finding out if they care or not. Fighting and provoking are my best talents. I'm not good at anything else."
>
> Consciously desperate for help, she started 5x weekly analysis, but her huge anxiety led to intense resistance. Terrified of separation and loss (though she denied this vehemently), she defended herself by not engaging with me or allowing herself to recognize any feelings of attachment. She often arrived 30 minutes late, or not at all, and was quite contemptuous of me. She announced, "Analysis is pointless

> anyway because I'm too crazy. Even a hundred Sigmund Freuds would never figure me out." I addressed her despair that she was irreparably damaged and mad, and interpreted her disappointment at being stuck with an ordinary therapist, not a celebrated "ideal": if she could not be perfect, she felt worthless; and if I wasn't Freud, I was useless. My struggle to contain my resentment and wish to retaliate was alleviated when I understood her dismissive behaviour *towards* me as an aggressively passive into active defence against feeling rejected *by* me. She was provoking me to test if I would reject and abandon her. Thinking of her aggression as like that of a panicky toddler in a tantrum helped me to regain my empathy. I interpreted her provocations as her wish to see if I could survive her attacks without rejecting her, as her wish to engage me in an exciting battle to ward-off feelings of depression and emptiness, and as her way of keeping control over the analysis for fear of being helplessly dependent on me. It soon became clear that her entrenched sado-masochistic style of relating provided a defence against core complex anxieties of abandonment and engulfment (Glasser, 1996), whereby she could maintain an optimal distance from, yet also a hold on the object. Her defiance towards her parents and me was reflected in an internal sado-masochistic battle between a punitive superego and her demanding and aggressive infantile wishes. Her aggression, directed towards others and herself via self-destructive and risk-taking behaviour, was insufficiently bound with loving feelings. She had no capacity for real concern—either for others or for herself. She felt spoilt by her parents "as if they don't care", and swung between a deeply self-denigrating self-image and a view of herself, imbued with bravado, as omnipotent and grandiose.

During adolescence, some risky behaviour is expectable as teenagers test their limits and 'try on' different types of identity, but (as with Lisa) risk-taking may represent an unresolved sense of omnipotence and the avoidance of independent mastery and self-care, developmental issues faced by the child in toddler-hood. A major developmental task of adolescence involves loosening the libidinal and aggressive ties to the parents in order to become an independent member of society. There are many reasons why an adolescent might be unable to detach in a healthy way from the parents, including unresolved ambivalence and aggression towards them. The adolescent may progress from suspiciousness of the parents to general paranoia. Or hostility and aggression may be deflected away from the parents and onto the self, leading to depression, self-denigration, self-harm and sometimes suicide.

Adolescence is a "normative crisis situation" (Tonnesmann, 1980) and a time of "developmental disturbance" when the typical fluctuations "between extreme opposites would be deemed highly abnormal at any other time of life" (A. Freud, 1980, p. 275). In the turmoil of adolescence, the young person's entire internal world is turned upside down. It is not surprising that they swing from wild excitement to deep depression and that their defences break down. Buxbaum wrote, "Just as the river, swollen with melting snow and torrential rains, breaks through its dams and floods the land, so the inordinately increased aggression floods the adolescent's whole system, explodes, and inundates society" (Buxbaum, 1970, p. 263). Delinquent and destructive enactments of aggression constitute the adolescent's rebellion not only against external authority but also, most importantly, against severe superego dictates. In the context of faulty superego development, guilt is unavailable as a signal and has to be defied and triumphed over.

Typical passions of the healthy adolescent concern matters of world importance—world peace, racism, animal rights—that are in their view treated complacently by the adult world. Such ideals provide a focus for directing adolescent aggression and passions in very adaptive and socially useful ways, whilst also allowing them to feel superior to the parents as they individuate from them. If the adolescent's earlier development has been good-enough, he will have established healthy modes of relating in which aggression is bound by loving and protective feelings so that aggression will be used for preservation of self and others and self-assertion. Physical aggression is sublimated through various hobbies, interests and skills, and channelled into activities such as competitive sports and verbal debate and, fused with loving feelings, into sexual activity. Language becomes the major medium for the expression of aggression, and in the relatively healthy adolescent this is confined to swearing and having the occasional row. The less healthy adolescent, who is still struggling to restrain his aggressive impulses, may be physically aggressive and will use words violently and destructively to vent his rage. This brings us back to the title of the paper.

Conclusion

I began with "biting teeth" and now end with "biting wit", both aspects of oral aggression. If biting wit takes the form of sarcasm, the destructiveness remains undisguised, unfunny and potentially damaging. If, however, it takes the form of irony (such as political satire), the aggressive content and intent is less directly destructive. Thus channelled, it can be a source of pleasurable fun as well as a means of communicating an ideological view.

The development of aggression is a massive topic. Some aspects mentioned perhaps deserve greater emphasis, but I have aimed to trace the main normative developmental issues and to emphasize some of the positive aspects of aggression as these tend to be given less attention in the literature. A concluding quote from Anna Freud reminds us that we all retain traces of aggression from every developmental level, and that throughout our lives we continue to struggle with them:

> . . . while libido and aggression move forward from one level to the next and cathect the objects which serve satisfaction on each stage, no station on the way is ever fully outgrown.
>
> [A. Freud, 1980, p. 95]

Note

1. This paper was previously published in Celia Harding (Ed.) (2006), *Aggression and Destructiveness: Psychoanalytic Perspectives*. London and New York: Routledge.

Acknowledgement

In fond memory of Rose Edgcumbe for her wisdom and clarity of mind.

CHAPTER EIGHT

Brief communications from the edge

Psychotherapy with challenging adolescents

Ann Horne

Prologue

The Winnicottian child, allowed an experience of "good-enough" in-tune mothering, is in a position to meet the world with confident curiosity. As a profession with different theoretical emphases in our trainings, we would hope equally as child psychotherapists to be able to greet each other with a similar curiosity—grounded in our own experience but engaging with the "other" with interest. In this area of work—with the adolescent who is on the cusp of a perverse or delinquent solution that may harden into character disorder—we need to be able to share ideas, think flexibly about what makes sense theoretically and what works clinically, and find an arena for sharing the burden of managing especially difficult counter-transferences (Winnicott, 1947; Lloyd-Owen, 1997; Wilson, 1999). Parsons and Dermen (1999), writing about the violent child and adolescent, describe this burden well:

> From the therapist's point of view, she has to deal with the impact of the child's very primitive anxieties which will inevitably trigger her own. In practice, the twin dangers are that she may either defend against her own anxieties by denying that she is with a patient who

> could well attack her, or be so afraid of this possibility that she cannot be receptive to the patient's needs . . . The patient will find it intolerable to be at the receiving end of the very defences upon which he relies . . . Additionally, the therapist will have to contend with the arousal of her sadism when attacked. She may respond to this by wishing to control or get rid of the patient. Since the work proceeds slowly and acting out is inevitable, she will also have to deal with feeling useless, helpless and guilty.
>
> [Parsons & Dermen, 1999, p. 344]

We may argue as to whether to interpret anxiety at once or not. When we do not do so, it is for the very good reason that interpreting such primitive anxiety too early in the analytic process may be counterproductive and simply strengthen maladaptive and perverse defences—a technical issue often elaborated by Anna Freud in her writings (A. Freud, 1936, pp. 36–37; 1968, p. 143). Indeed, in sustaining traditional and often fundamentalist theoretical positions, rather than engaging with curiosity with each other, we can attack each other with theoretical and technical difference, not recognizing in our rigidity and our activity that we actually mirror the defences of the challenging adolescent.

The challenging adolescent, who if an adult would attract a forensic label, has *not* found a position of confident curiosity in relation to his world. Where early trauma, overwhelming to the immature ego and not able to be processed, has been a feature (as it frequently has), the young person has often been left with early body-centred defences as a way of blocking out the primitive anxieties of annihilation, abandonment, disintegration, falling endlessly and merging. In the therapy room we encounter in the patient and ourselves the capacity to act in and out, and experience anxiety about acting-out outside—when society may well intervene. As Winnicott (1963a) notes:

> . . . the analyst must expect to find acting-out in the transference, and must understand the significance of this acting-out, and be able to give it positive value.
>
> [Winnicott, 1963a, p. 210]

In the counter-transference we find ourselves in touch with fundamental primitive fears, cruel and punishing superegos, immature atoll-like egos, and defences designed to deny intimacy, attachment, affect and pain. We need to cope with not-knowing—often for long spells—and to think both developmentally and psychoanalytically (Alvarez, 1996; Fonagy & Target, 1996), recognizing when the opportunity of becoming a "new object" glimmers, yet in touch with the dangers inherent in this for the patient (Loewald, 1960).

Introducing Matthew

Matthew was 14 years old when he abused the 7-year-old sister of a friend. The court requested, through the Youth Justice Social Worker, an assessment as to the suitability of psychotherapy for Matthew in relation to his offence. I saw him three times around his fifteenth birthday, a colleague meeting his paternal grandmother and stepmother and then his father and stepmother. Once-weekly therapy began two months later.

Matthew's parents married when his mother was 17 and his father 18, his mother being 6 months pregnant with Matthew. Matthew's mother had been brought up in an abusive home and was sexually and physically abused by her stepfather as well as suffering severe emotional neglect. Her mother had died when Matthew's mother was 13 year old. Mr P (Matthew's father) had suffered serious depression from his early teens, attempting suicide twice and having a spell of adolescent in-patient psychiatric treatment. He had, according to his own mother, suffered most in the family when his parents separated when he was 4 years old. When Matthew was 3 years old, his father's depression worsened and Matthew's mother ended their relationship. Mr P moved in with his mother, Matthew's grandmother who came to the clinic. His wife moved a boyfriend, Sean, into the home with Matthew and her. There were violent episodes between the parents which occurred because of Mr P's requests for access to Matthew, and an injunction was granted by the court that banned Mr P from approaching the home. He spent a few weeks in prison, having destroyed their kitchen, and did not see his son for over a year.

Sean disliked Matthew. It was only following the referral that Sean's gross physical abuse of Matthew emerged as the family started to be able to talk of it. Matthew knows that this relationship was abusive but has blocked out his memory of it. He does, however, recall his parents arguing and fighting.

When Matthew was five, his mother was killed in a road traffic accident—she was knocked down by a car on a zebra crossing. Matthew was left in the "care" of his abuser as his mother had stated that this was her wish in her will. There ensued a long custody battle, Matthew being made a Ward of Court and, at one point when he had been sent to stay with his abusive maternal step-grandfather, he was kidnapped by his father and grandmother, so anxious were they about his care. Matthew's father finally won custody. When Matthew was 6½, he and his father moved in with Mr P's girlfriend, Sammie, and her daughter, Emma, who is a year younger than Matthew. They now have a son, Alex, who is 11 years younger than Matthew.

Matthew's past and present functioning

Mr P and Sammie approached their local Child and Family Consultation Service when Matthew was 7 years old, for help with his aggression, but it was felt that time to adjust to the new family was all that was needed. By the age of nine, Matthew had been expelled from six schools, sometimes for violence, sometimes for not being there. He described escaping out of school windows and commented, "I thought that was mad—being expelled for not even being there!" There was no sense of a comprehending or a pursuing adult. Finally he ended up in a day school for children with emotional and behavioural difficulties, a school that creditably managed to hold on to him.

In school he was said to be "bright"—brighter than most of his peers, "capable of clear thinking but stubborn". He could attack other children with words, and be rude, unpleasant and undermining to others. This verbal aggression remained worrying to the school and it tipped over into physical fights at perceived slights.

Peer relations were said to be poor by school and family, although it emerged in therapy that Matthew belonged to a group of delinquent lads with whom he spent much of his spare time. His descriptions of their meetings contained much excitement and activity, and were empty of thought or reflection. Matthew had an ambivalent relationship with his father whom he tried to like but who shouted at him, hit him and only rarely listened. He could have been allied to his stepmother, Sammie, as both are intelligent, but he felt excluded by the birth of his half brother, Alex. His paternal grandmother remained a "good object" for him.

His offence occurred when he was at a friend's watching England being beaten by Argentina in the World Cup. This friend often had sexual intercourse with his girlfriend in the presence of a group of friends, which Matthew found exciting and disturbing. When he went to the toilet, his friend's seven-year-old little sister pounced on him from her bedroom to play, punching him and jumping on his back, and he threw her onto her bed. There he began to tickle her and what began as a game moved to his touching her genitals. When he found that he was trying to remove her pants, he stopped himself, wondered what he was doing, and went home. The others in the family, however, had a sense of something more sinister and later in the evening asked the little girl what had happened. Matthew was arrested at 2 a.m. and taken to the police station. He told me his father followed but, in fact, it was Sammie who came to see him. Initially insistently denying everything, when faced finally with the video interview with the child he agreed that her version was right. He received a 3-year Supervision Order, with a strong injunction from the judge that, should he appear in court on any count in future, he would be given a custodial sentence. When I saw him he was embarrassed to talk of it and ashamed of what he had done—hopeful signs. Like many violated young people, however, he was furious that the police had kept his clothes for analysis—as if he were trying to focus on the external to avoid thinking of the body, its actions and the internal.

Thinking about work with adolescents

The key tasks of adolescence, as we all know, involve separation, individuation and becoming responsible for the self. In classical theory where psychosexual development is the main thrust, this means taking ownership of the body and sexuality at a time of great change. Where there has been early trauma and the immature ego has been overwhelmed, we have to think with care about technique. Defences are often pre-verbal, pre-representational, centring on the body-self, its traumatization and its survival. What the young person does *with* the body, therefore, is significant:

1. in the offence of sexually abusing others (the victim's report is extremely helpful in letting us know just what is so intolerable that it has to be decanted outside the self);

2. in delinquency and putting the body at risk;
3. in violence or aggression where we often encounter either violent provocation designed to repeat an earlier experience of being violated, or self-preservative violence in Glasser's (1998) terms, designed to protect the fragile ego from perceived threat;
4. in the unconscious use of the body in ensuring one's exploitation. The prime example of this is the rent boy whose repetition-compulsion in relation to his own abuse is masked by a veneer of being in control of those whom he chooses to think he seduces and who are made to "pay".

Thus issues around the body, bodily conflicts and its use need to be addressed. Yet the adolescent task is to take over this body at a time when infantile fantasy and curiosity is revived. One solution for the therapist is to separate mind and body—"Isn't it interesting what your body gets up to—being chased, being hit, being where it shouldn't be?" Addressing the functioning part to explore together the infantile part can help "save face" and avoid humiliation. Sometimes, though, this is not enough. Edgcumbe (1988) approached such issues when thinking about the technical problems of interpreting (or not) in the transference with adolescents, and "whether to take up defence, content or affect, and at what depth or level to deal with content of conflicts" in the light of "the adolescent's heightened fear and shame about regression . . ." (Edgcumbe 1988, p. 1). Following case illustrations, she concludes:

> I have stressed the importance of taking up material from the angle of the higher level conflicts which have engendered regression, rather than the infantile instinctual wishes and modes of relating which are expressed in the regression . . . Shame and anxiety are likely to be best relieved by making sense of the situation which led to the regression. In this way the analyst can remain aligned with the part of the patient's self which is striving for growth, without denying the regression.
>
> [*ibid.*, p. 12]

It is just this kind of carefully thought-out, conscious choice of what to take up that often seems to have been totally misunderstood in the past in disputes between theoretical traditions. It led Winnicott in 1962 to an interim, transitional position that he called "working as a psychoanalyst" when the "anti-social tendency" (amongst other clinical issues) was present. Today, one hopes, we are clearer that this *is* psychotherapy and that it is, moreover, a question of conscious, sophisticated analytic choice.

In parallel with issues about the body comes the danger of relationships and especially of intimacy. Of particular importance in work with young people in search of a perverse solution (a survival technique) is Glasser's (1979; 1996) concept of the core complex. Here, one sees the search for intimacy as the start of what becomes a vicious circle. Gaining intimacy, the adolescent is overwhelmed by anxieties of a primitive nature—anxiety about merging with the object, of suffocation and loss of individuation. This arouses a violent response—violence in the service of protecting the immature ego—in order to escape anxiety; and a consequent sense of abandonment (again, a primitive anxiety) ensues with the necessity once more to pursue intimacy. And "la ronde" continues. Glasser finds this to underlie all perverse psychopathology.

Psychotherapy requires a relationship of considerable intimacy, yet the adolescent process, too, is contrary to this. Apart from the danger in hoping that this relationship might be different from earlier ones, the adolescent can experience being understood both as a relief and as an enormous threat, bringing back just such primitive fears of merging with the object, of not being separate. One has to *pace* this experience of being understood and be aware of what is too intimate, and know that the young person may be driven to disparage it when it is desired, arousing as it does memories of vulnerability. Even pauses and silence need judgement: silence may become a threatening absence of the object, especially if this mirrors the young person's early life. At times, one has to be an "enlivening object" (Alvarez 1992); otherwise one is perceived as abandoning and annihilating. It is "either–or": there is little middle ground here—indeed, the process of therapy seeks to develop this. The "all or nothing" quality Winnicott encapsulates in "There is not yet a capacity to identify with parent figures without loss of personal identity" (Winnicott, 1963b, p. 244) is exacerbated in the adolescent who has still to achieve a capacity for symbolization, for whom emotional states *are* bodily experiences (Parsons & Dermen, 1999, p. 341). The risk involved in "hope", too, may be one reason why, with adolescents, one often gets "brief communications" followed by escape.

We are all used to adolescents as escapologists. In a sense, this is a healthy adolescent process, distancing oneself. It contains elements of the toddler who has learned how to make the adults pursue him—except that with adolescents we are made to feel great uncertainty as to how much we should pursue. This capacity to put the grown-up into a "double bind" seems to arrive with the hormones at puberty. Again, this requires delicacy: the conflict belongs in the adolescent, not in the therapist or network, and should be gently returned there. A very simple example would be the adolescent who invariably arrives 15 minutes late for his session. One can say how important taking control is, and how essential; it is a pity, however, that in taking this necessary step he costs himself 15 minutes of *his* time. That's an interesting dilemma he has there—and the conflict is quietly returned to its owner but not in the tone of his own dismissive and shaming superego. The other side of escapology is the defence of activity—a return to the body-self of toddler years. Activity often occurs as a way of blocking out thought, which itself involves unbearable recollection and memory. It is, in this context, unfortunate that the UK Government has instructed the Probation Service in England and Wales to breach offenders (i.e., to bring them back before the Court) if they miss two appointments. One could point to recourse to action and an absence of thought in Government for this anti-adolescent decision. Thinking, too, in adolescence is a further aspect of intimacy—intimacy of mind—and

> The fear of thinking may derive both from conflicts over curiosity and from reluctance to let the analyst/mother intrude on painful private matters. Here, again, transference interpretation may have to be used sparingly, to free the patient's thinking.
>
> [Edgcumbe, 1988, p. 13]

Creating a space for thought is not easy when the drive is to activity and not thinking. Making space for curiosity about the self helps, and one can often capture adolescents by picking up the paradoxes in their lives or offering the unexpected in comment, especially when the unexpected is in contrast to their dismissive, abandoning or punitive superego:

> Matthew described being on the back of a friend's motorbike (legitimately) in the park and the police cruising past. By their actions, the group made the police pursue them, but eluded them. I said that was interesting. Matthew had expected something more negative. "How?" I said that he had really made the police pay attention. Perhaps he had wished people had done so when he was little. Matthew went on to say how his father often thought he was "up to something" when he was not, then told of his favourite teacher, a female Art teacher, who had taken his side in a dispute that he had actually caused, leading to another youth being punished. He grinned. I said that perhaps I needed to hear the warning—all is not necessarily as it seems? He grinned more widely. I said that this was another area for me to be curious about—he can change reality.

It is worth thinking here about the concept of "therapist as developmental object", so well described by Hurry (1998) and a part of the work of the Hampstead Clinic for many years. The young person engages with a curious ego and supportive superego in the "developmental object therapist" who *deliberately* takes up a position of *not* being used as a projection of the child's cruel, shaming and undermining superego. When one thinks of early trauma and the "breaching of the shame shield" described by Campbell (1994) in the young abusers whom he has treated over 30 years, one sees a further reason for creating possibilities for alternative identifications and routes to a different ego ideal. Wilson (1999), writing about delinquents, put it rather well:

> The key therapeutic task is to resist the young person's implicit invitation to repeat the past . . . The . . . ability to find ways of responding that are different from what young people expect and which do not meet the dictates of the transference is essential. Ultimately, it is through the child psychotherapists' behaviour that they convey their understanding of the meaning of the young person's delinquency and provide the safety and boundary that the delinquent needs. Such

> behaviour, sustained by the child psychotherapists' own insights, constitutes interpretation and serves as a stimulus and basis for further verbal forms of communication and understanding.
>
> [Wilson, 1999, p. 318]

It is also important, with the drive to acting-out in adolescence and the risk of self-harm, that there is a functioning network that enables the therapy to continue, a subject addressed later.

Issues of sexuality appear throughout the treatment, often beginning in the form of remarkably crude jokes that show very early childish fantasies of destruction, inadequacy and incorporation in intercourse. The fantasies of adolescence, after all, overlay for such young people a very often traumatically abusive childhood reality. Work in this area tends, I find, to be consolidated nearer the end of treatment although it appears throughout—it is only after much work that the young person can, with confidence, face exploring the kind of adult sexual being that they would wish to be, and the fears and fantasies around that. Issues of a procreative body are acute for abusing and violated boys and girls. The necessary fusion of aggression, agency and sexuality for adult functioning is terrifying in its potential for destruction and much work on the positive role of aggression is necessary first.

Young people, defending against the memory of helplessness in the absence of a protective object, find aggression paradoxically difficult. It emerges in an uncontrollable fashion in their lives, overwhelming others and themselves. They need practice in appropriately assertive aggression and righteous anger, and a capacity to recognize and name emotions and affects, in order not to be swamped by them. Identifying with the adolescent's victim role can mean the therapist missing aggression: it is important to have in mind as a constant undercurrent, and to connote aggression and agency as necessary and, where it is problematic, to perceive the roots in an early defence against intolerable feelings. "Anger management" strategies work well where there is a more integrated, functioning "self"; where this is not so, the construction of an emotional vocabulary and "anger practice"—the capacity to recognize agency and aggression, to note when they are appropriate and to begin to exercise them—are essential. Attention to such ego developments as affect recognition and affect tolerance is vital in psychoanalytic work with young people where the ego is immature and like patchwork.

There are implications within all of this for assessment—the information one needs, the environment necessary for an assessment to be relevant and if therapy is to be considered, and the assessment encounter itself. These are beyond the remit of this paper but must be flagged up: "The essential thing is I do base my work on diagnosis," said Winnicott to the British Psycho-analytic Society (Winnicott, 1962, p. 169).

Thinking about Matthew

Matthew presents as not typical of young abusers but rather demonstrating the mixed symptomatology of mid-adolescents who arouse concern. Most abusing adolescents appear either to be rather isolated individuals with one clear *known* abusive incident, or to be multiple abusers with a real polymorphous feel. Matthew's history shows difficulties in equal peer relations (his mates are all less bright than he is), long-standing outbursts of aggression and seeking violent situations, delinquency and sexual abusing. His capacity for putting himself at risk is also becoming clearer.

With Matthew we can see the clear pattern of early violence where there is no protective figure, outlined in the Great Ormond Street Hospital research on young abusers: the two main factors correlating with abusing others are:

1. an experience of unpredictable and unprocessable violence and trauma, when the ego is too immature to make sense of it (Lanyado *et al.*, 1995). Matthew witnessed early marital warfare, was beaten from the age of three and traumatically abandoned to his abuser at age five;
2. having a mother who has herself been abused and unconsciously projects onto her male child the expectation that he, too, will abuse.

The memory of such victimization (especially the humiliation and vulnerability) can be dealt with by developing a fantasy of abusing someone weaker and smaller, becoming powerful in the process and making someone else into the victim—identification with the aggressor. Part of the treatment thus involves exploring the patient's own "victim" experience before one can reach the victimizing.

There is also "the ambivalence of the object"—a mother who consciously and deliberately leaves him with an abuser—and who turns a blind eye to his abuse when she is there. We should not be surprised that he "tricks" the grown-ups in return and should expect this in the therapy. Thinking inter-generationally, Matthew's mother was abused and abandoned on her mother's death to her abuser and the scenario was repeated with Matthew. Matthew's father lost his father at age 4; his mother lost her natural father at a very young age; Matthew lost his for a considerable spell at age 3. Welldon (1988) has alerted us to the necessity of thinking across at least three generations where abuse is concerned.

We can also note the use of activity as a defence, beginning with his early escaping from school—but no-one pursues, instead he unconsciously makes the process of his being abandoned happen repeatedly—and continuing in his delinquency. Indeed, one might find his delinquent activities to be a seduction of me, as therapist, away from the abusing that formed his offence, as well as a practised way of using excitement to mask depression. There is also the compulsion to repeat sensations of fear, as we will see in the clinical material: in some of his delinquent activities, Matthew scares himself. More profoundly, one might think about identification with the dead mother: it is unusual for a 22-year-old to have made a will and colleagues have suggested that her accident may have been suicide. Being alert as to Matthew's unconscious "suicidal" behaviour, therefore, becomes a factor, and the meaning of an abandoning, not protective, even malevolent maternal object is important.

Finally, it is worth commenting on aggression, an issue of long standing for Matthew, noted first at the age of 7. This use of self-preservative violence has begun to turn into an enjoyment of others getting into trouble—the early beginnings of a sadistic quality—and it is essential for his development that work is done with Matthew on this.

An encounter with Matthew

This session occurred in early December, almost 9 months into therapy. Matthew at this point is living with his grandmother.

Matthew arrived early for his session, wearing a new, padded, warm jacket. (He had come the previous week in a sweatshirt and with an awful cold.) Although his cold was still bad, he said that he was OK, that he had taken lots of soup. This comment came with a smile—in our last session he had told me that his grandmother was very good at making soup. (Paternal grandmother has transference implications.) He hadn't been allowed to take a day off school, however. I wondered if he could have been able to bear that—not being active and just sitting with his thoughts. He agreed he could not; he would rather be in school. I reflected on this unusually intimate start and wondered when reaction would set in. (When Matthew attends, he always takes time to re-discover his object: he seems, indeed, to expect a corrupt object.)

There was a sustained pause. He looked very sad. I wondered if he were thoughtful now or just fed up? Fed up. His father had said that the moped was too much for his Christmas present and he probably wouldn't get it. He expanded on how it would have cost £200. His father was giving his brother Alex a computer worth £200; Matthew would get a new mobile phone worth £100 and his sister, Emma, a present worth £75. There was a pause, half sad, half angry. I wondered rather weakly if that seemed unfair? *Yes*—Alex gets everything. (Alex, indulged at age 5, contrasts with Matthew, abused and abandoned.)

After a further pause Matthew wondered if his father would give him the money and he could put it towards a bike himself. Then he deflated, recalling that his father preferred to pay things up week by week. I said that it seemed impossible for the adults to get things right for him. We reflected in silence.

"Do you know a Pa . . . Po . . .—something like that—it's a bike." It emerged as a Piaggio. "They're *very* nice! I really like them. I was out last night on one!" I felt anxiety begin to rise and wondered inside about this need to make the adult anxious, and why. There followed a story of Matthew and five or six friends. Dave had brought the bike and all had tried it out in the local park. Steve did a "wheelie" and drove into a tree. Matthew also tried it—"It was really good!" He described sharp turns, sudden acceleration, mud flying, excitement. As he was in full flow, his mobile phone rang. He looked apologetic, muttered, "Sorry", said the answering service would pick it up, and could not resist checking the screen. It was Dave leaving a message: "He already phoned twice when I was on the train coming here! It's about meeting tonight." The phone was switched off and put away. He continued with the bike tale—taking it out on the road out of town, a vivid description of Dave nearly coming off the back of the bike as Matthew accelerated, "It can do 45 miles an hour!" and finally return to town.

I thought about the sense of life and energy in the midst of this extremely dangerous behaviour. "You know, you really like being 'on the edge', don't you." Matthew looked questioning. I said that on the bike he liked being in control himself (he didn't like being on the back) but it could tip over—Steve had managed to hit a tree. I suggested he was also "on the edge" with the police, were he found, and with the court as the judge had told him that his return to court on any count would mean a custodial sentence. And he had told me before (in an earlier session) that being on a bike could be scary and he didn't like that. "Yes, that's why I won't let Steve drive."

There was a pause. I interpreted then that it was interesting that this "on the edge" excitement had actually followed a very painful description of him and Emma feeling "on the edge" in the family. He gave me a very direct look. I offered that one way he had learned of being in control of these very difficult, sad feelings was through the excited "on the edge" feelings, but they were risky. I wondered, too, about the excitement keeping *me* "on the edge", not sure of his safety, and wondered if he was good at making the adults and me feel this. He smiled gently.

There was quite a long pause. Matthew launched into a story of his friend, Joseph, a very small 14-year-old. Joseph's passion was cars—with a particular emphasis on taking and driving them away. I noted to myself the connection between my interpretation of the pain in the family and his further recourse to excitement and danger, moving from bikes to cars, but did not interrupt. Matthew gave great detail of how Joseph would break into the black boxes behind the steering wheel panel, where to locate these in a Rover Metro, and diverted into a variety of ways to break into a car. Joseph had been doing this since he was 7 years old. The police knew him well—had been to see him the other day as he is the first port of call when cars go missing. "He has been cautioned and the police know him. Pathetic!" "Pathetic—who?" I asked. "Joe. He knows they'll come to see him first. When he takes a car he drives with the headlights on full beam so that he can't be seen himself. He just gets very excited by cars. Once when

I was with him he saw a Jaguar. I said, '*No!*' but Joe kept talking about what it would be like to drive it when we were walking away." I wondered if Joe had the same sense of excitement in relation to cars that Matthew had talked of with bikes. He looked surprised: "No, he's pathetic." I commented that sometimes things are both pathetic and exciting, reminding him of the 36-inch television set he said his father had bought that in one way seemed pathetic to him but in another seemed full of excitement and potential. This had been in an earlier session. He grinned—"That's true!" I continued, "So you know some things that are both pathetic—daft—dangerous and pathetic—exciting—'on the edge'?" He nodded thoughtfully.

The story of Joe continued. He had "torched" a car. This felt suddenly very unsafe, as if the juxtaposition of "pathetic" and "excitement" had to be avoided. He had tried to break into a car in Tesco's car park (the known area where local youth find and dump cars and bikes) but couldn't get at the black box. Realizing that he had left his fingerprints all over the vehicle, he had found a cloth and jerrycan of petrol in the boot and poured it over the front seats, leaving the can in the car before striking a match. He had singed his hair. "He's totally pathetic! He could have burned himself badly. He had the rag from the boot—he could have wiped off his fingerprints. He ran off and it went 'Whump!' exploding. The Fire Brigade was called. He could have hurt people!" Matthew sounded very upset. I said gently that I thought he had witnessed this, been there with Joe. He nodded. I added that it was frightening that the excitement and "on the edge" bits could tip right over into danger and wondered if he scared himself. He nodded, saying, "He could have been harmed!" Yes. After a pause I added that it was interesting that such a memory of danger had followed my saying to him that he wanted me to feel "on the edge" sometimes—that he was letting me know how dreadfully dangerous things sometimes felt for him and that it was right that we were both concerned.

He recalled a teacher at school, in car mechanics class, whom Matthew had asked something that implied how to hot-wire cars. The teacher had given him the information and not asked why he wanted to know. I said I thought he was letting me know about two things. Firstly, grown-ups may not be straight but collude with exciting illegal things, like the teacher giving him the information. (I was thinking of corrupt objects again.) How, then, could he possibly know to trust me and my concern? Secondly, perhaps he was warning me that he could be tricky—tricking the teacher and perhaps other grown-ups, like me. He gave me a very direct, straight look.

Collusion, of course, is one of the major pressures felt in the counter-transference with psychopathic patients (Symington, 1980).

There was a further pause. Matthew said, "The bike engine's still running." The bike, of course, had been stolen and hot-wired. His friends were "second time thieves", having come across it stolen and abandoned. They had by-passed the ignition and could not turn off the engine. They would have to cover the exhaust pipe, cutting off the air supply. (All endings, I thought, are traumatic—even for the bike.) "Someone stole it last night." I must have looked astonished. "Yeah, when we'd gone home Dave had left it at his back gate and phoned to say it had been taken. We found Steve had taken it and had it at his place. It would have been pathetic if a nicked bike had been nicked—I mean we couldn't report it to the police, could we?" I said that I thought that was really interesting: that, when something has gone wrong in the past, the grown-ups will simply not take a young person seriously. Perhaps in some ways this was a little like Matthew—it is impossible for him to hope that the adults will be concerned *now* for his safety when they made such a bad job of it in the past. "You mean Sean," said Matthew, referring to his mother's abusive boyfriend. "Yes, and everything that happened then. Now, as a result of that, you are making me into another of these grown-ups who hears very dangerous things but can't stop you. Sometimes it feels better to do that than for you to hope that it might be different."

The following pause felt more thoughtful. "I'll only go tonight if Steve has a crash helmet for me. I know he's got one. It *is* scary—but exciting scary." ("Crash helmet" has become equated with me, interesting when one thinks about heads and minds.) I added that that was why he insists on driving, being in control: "It's like not taking the risk that the adults won't protect you again, but it's also the same 'on the edge' excitement of waiting for something to happen that was awful and too much for you when you were little." Matthew nodded slowly.

It was almost time to stop. Matthew checked the clock and put on his jacket. He told me that he *was* careful as sometimes it could get too scary. Moreover tonight they wouldn't be on the road but in a farmer's field. I said that he was taking on some of the adult bits about protecting himself but still being "on the edge". He was leaving me with something to worry about—perhaps he needed to do that. He gave a quiet smile and "See you next week!" I thought it was a promise to stay alive.

A note on networks

There must be a functioning, communicating network that is able to create a safe, holding structure if therapy for the young person who is a risk to himself and/or others is to be considered a treatment of choice. We all recall Winnicott's exhortation that delinquents need placement, not psychoanalysis, after he had the clinic basement flooded, his car jump-started and his buttocks bitten—more than once—by his first child analytic patient (Winnicott, 1956; 1963a). If there is not such a network, the issue is certainly placement. One could view this as offering practical "containers" until the stage is reached where words can contain and anxiety be symbolized rather than enacted. This cannot be stressed enough. Our omnipotence—or pressure from the network—may take us into a therapeutic relationship that then fails because external containment and understanding are lacking, and we repeat and re-visit trauma upon a young person who unconsciously seeks it. In Matthew's case the problems of finding a good residential community did not arise. There was a functioning, thinking network: he was at a good EBD school, had a three-year Supervision Order from the court, which gave time to work, and had a good, involved social worker. His family moved a distance away but, with joint planning, Matthew stayed with his grandmother through the week, sustaining attendance at the same school, and went to his father at weekends. Issues arose about leaving school: this is often experienced by adolescents as the school's abandonment of them, although they cannot articulate this, and the temptation is to get oneself thrown out or to leave it before it leaves you. This Matthew tried—and the network contained. He completed his exams.

It is also important that the network be experienced as safe and "holding" as, in therapy, the young person will inevitably get in touch with the early feelings of victimization and humiliation that led to the offending behaviour. Such a time may present a risk of suicide—as does the later stage when the adolescent begins to look at what he has done to others and guilt and shame arise—and a good support structure is essential. Equally, the defences, based on activity, may reassert themselves, as they did originally, to blot out such pain and the risk of further offending ensues. This has to be understood and *not* reacted to in a superego-ish way.

Networks suffer transference and counter-transference processes. All too often, this remains unconscious and damaging. It is *vital*, when working with young perpetrators, that a "case manager" be appointed to work with the network and help the unconscious become conscious. This needs an experienced person.

When warfare breaks out in the network, or communication stops and unilateral decision-making appears, there seem to be three main processes at work (Horne 1999):

1. Individuals in the network identify with and take up the positions of different family members (Kolvin & Trowell 1996). Such identifications polarize—the young person is either viewed as a poor traumatized victim or seen as a dangerous perpetrator; the parents are said to be overwhelmed by their ungrateful evil child or perceived as dreadfully neglectful and abusive. Holding all views together and recognizing the transference manifestations is vital.
2. The family system also gets re-enacted in the network—the myths, collusions and strategies for family homeostasis become replayed by all of us.
3. The internal world of the offender patient is realized in the network where we repeat the functions and attitudes of internal objects and "willingly" reinforce unhelpful defences (Davies 1996), principally the drive to activity. This compulsion to act, to *do something*, is commonplace and, as therapists, we will enrage other services at times by refusing to do this but requesting space to think together. The process of by-passing thought and reflection, after all, is the delinquent and abusing adolescent's prime defence, and he unconsciously tries to make it ours.

There is a paradigm from Transactional Analysis that is very helpful when thinking of networks. It comprises a triangle:

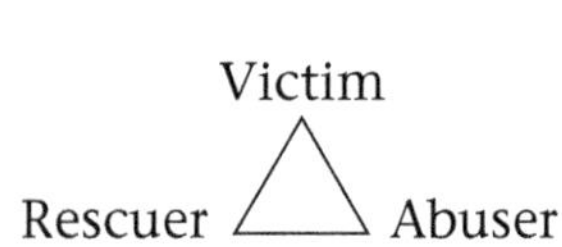

We move around it, not at will but pushed by others, taking up all positions. It is a salutary blow to one's omnipotence to be brought in as a "rescuer", but quickly to be defined by the network as an "abuser" (of the child by keeping him in therapy; of colleagues by not being able to say that he is no longer a risk)—and one becomes a victim oneself.

Conclusion

Keeping grounded and keeping sane are the two main tasks for the worker with acting-out adolescents. Regular clinical discussion is essential, both for support and survival but also to ensure that we are not seeing only one part of the young person or complying with "the dictates of the transference" (Wilson, 1999). A colleague can provide an Oedipal third for reflection, an antidote to primitive pre-Oedipal defences and anxieties. Pace and intimacy are important technical issues, and the level at which to take up conflicts (Edgcumbe, 1988) is an important aspect of judging these. The impact of developmental deficit, body-based defences and preverbal trauma should inform our assessment and work, and a developmental and psychoanalytic framework is essential. Most importantly, "thought, not action" is the key for patient and psychotherapist—creating space for thinking and reflection.

Epilogue

A year on, Matthew's "delinquent group" is now a social group. All are in work and the group now includes girls—opening up issues of sexuality in therapy. A sense of responsibility is a strong feature of his functioning. He dared to ask if there might be any flexibility when he is in work—could I still see him but at a later time?—a big risk, to ask for something, and on my letting him know that this was possible he promptly missed the next session (a telephone call—"I've lost my train fare!"). Intimacy still takes careful negotiation.

Note

This chapter was presented at the ACP Conference in September 2000. Earlier versions were given at conferences in Prague, Surrey and London. I am grateful to all these colleagues for helpful feedback and ideas.

This chapter was previously published in *Journal of Child Psychotherapy*, 2001, *27*(1): 3–18 (published by Routledge).

Acknowledgement

I am especially grateful to two Portman colleagues—Marianne Parsons and Dorothy Lloyd-Owen—and to Monica Lanyado for their generosity with time, discussion and thought, and to the Portman team who always respond with creativity to child and adolescent clinical presentations.

CHAPTER NINE

Compulsive use of virtual sex and internet pornography

Addiction or perversion?

Heather Wood

"Virtual sex" has many forms; internet pornography, telephone sex chatlines and "chatting" online or texting sexually explicit messages may all be used as sexual stimuli. These activities are deemed "virtual" because although they entail imagined scenarios where there may be a fantasy of other participants, actually the person is alone and the sexual act consists of masturbation; in addition, the term "virtual" refers to the use of new media technologies to access sexually stimulating materials to elaborate or reflect the person's fantasy. The use of sexually explicit materials to stimulate sexual fantasy and masturbation is not new and is not in itself a problem; people often seek help at the point when the behaviour has become frequent, compulsive and distressing, and appears to jeopardize or impair other intimate relationships or to impinge on the individual's working life. For those accessing illegal pornography (i.e. child pornography) there are added concerns for the individual about detection, arrest and criminal conviction, and for others about the exploitation and abuse of the children depicted in the imagery.

Within the literature and within clinical practice, the compulsive use of internet pornography is the predominant focus of concern and apparently the most pervasive problem. However, I want to broaden this out and address the various forms of "virtual sex" interchangeably. There may be something very specific about the power of visual imagery and looking in the use of pornography, but, with respect to the kinds of issues discussed here, there do not appear to be qualitative differences between the person who looks at pornography, and those compulsively using phone chat-lines, or those who use the internet or mobile phones to exchange sexually explicit messages while masturbating.

It has been observed that pornography is always a front-runner in exploiting new media technologies. Within the last year patients have started to talk about the use of web-cams so that they can now see and be seen by the person they are interacting with online; downloading pornography from the internet to their mobile phones; and of people accessing pornography through someone else's wireless connection to evade detection. Within the next year, no doubt, such things will either have become commonplace or eclipsed by still more ingenious methods of exploiting developments in the technology.

There are statistics which give us some indication of the pervasiveness of virtual sex and the proportion of people for whom it has become problematic. It has been suggested that almost 70 per cent of all dollars spent online are spent on sexual pursuits (Sprenger, 1999 cited in Cooper Griffin-Shelley, 2002). A recent article in the *Guardian* newspaper in the UK (Aitkenhead, 2006) referred to an estimate by British Telecom that 100,000 people attempt to access child pornography on the internet every day. If the adult male population of Britain is about 20 million people, and assuming this activity is mainly restricted to men, this would be approximately one in 200 men. A review of a number of large sample studies of the use of "virtual sexuality in the workplace" suggests that 20 per cent of respondents used the internet for sexual activities while at work (Cooper, McLoughlin and Campbell, 2000). Greenfield (1999) conducted a survey of 17,251 respondents and concluded that 6 per cent were internet addicted, and of these 20 per cent were sexually addicted, suggesting that a little over 1 per cent of internet users may develop an addiction to online sexual activity. When the number of people accessing the internet worldwide is now counted in billions (clickz.com estimate 1.08 billion worldwide in 2005 and a projected figure of 1.8 billion by 2010), and the number of active users in the UK (using the internet at least once a month) is estimated to be 24.36 million (clickz.com), the number in difficulty must be very considerable.

In 1996 and 1997 there were no referrals to the Portman Clinic for compulsive use of internet pornography. In 1998 we received just one. By 2003 it had become one of the most common problems cited in referral and assessment information, alongside paedophilia, transvestism and assault. For the referral year to March 2003, on the basis of referral and assessment information, this was identified as a problem in 11 per cent of all referred adult patients (Wood, Ramadhan & Delmar-Morgan, 2005).

It is striking that very little has been written about the use of internet technology from a psychoanalytic point of view, with Gabbard's (2001) account of the use of e-mail by a patient to express an erotic transference to her therapist before this could be acknowledged within the consulting room and Young's (1996; 1998; 2003) internet-published papers as notable exceptions.

The literature on compulsive use of internet pornography, or cybersex as the Americans tend to call it, is almost entirely American, and almost entirely coined within an addiction model. The individual is seen to be in the grip of a behavioural addiction, and treatment focuses on strengthening motivation and strategies of self-management to reduce repetitive and compulsive behaviour and to foster alternative coping strategies and sources of gratification (see for example Delmonico, Griffin, & Carnes, 2002). Such approaches may include some consideration of the underlying function of the behaviour and its significance in terms of personal history; Delmonico, Griffin and Carnes (2002), for example, include "understanding the dynamics and decision processes of the sexually intrusive behaviour" and "understanding family of origin/childhood trauma issues" in their "sample cybersex treatment plan" (pp. 157–158). However, the way that this is presented implies that it would not extend to a full psychoanalytic understanding. Perhaps as a reflection of the underlying model of sexually compulsive behaviours, a group of respected American clinicians are lobbying to have sexual addiction included in DSM IV as one of the category of behavioural addictions, along with gambling

(Carnes, 2000). In parallel with this, it is striking how often patients present referring to their addiction.

The addiction model is undoubtedly of value. It has "face validity", addressing the patient's sense of being in the grip of something compulsive and addictive, and it no doubt generates useful, focussed treatment strategies. However, I think that the addiction model may be used defensively, and that this defence may be used by patients and clinicians alike, to turn a blind eye to the meaning of the behaviours. Specifically, I think it turns a blind eye to the perverse aspects of these behaviours.

The term "perversion" has moral connotations. Definitions in the *Shorter Oxford English Dictionary* include "turning aside from truth or right; diversion to an improper use; corruption, distortion". In the diagnostic field the term has been replaced by the morally more neutral "paraphilia". DSM IV (American Psychiatric Association, 2000), for example, stipulates that the key characteristics of paraphilias are recurrent, intense sexually-arousing fantasies, sexual urges or behaviours, usually involving either non-human objects, the suffering or humiliation of oneself or one's partner, or children or non-consenting persons. The paraphilic fantasies or stimuli may be used episodically or may be perceived to be essential to sexual arousal, but must have an enduring role within the psyche and be used over a period of 6 months or more. Psychoanalysts would also stress these characteristics, viewing perversions as fixed, repetitive compulsive sexual behaviours or fantasies, which may not be essential to the sexual act but may be necessary to experience a subjective sense of full satisfaction. However, psychoanalysts continue to use the term perversion, not to pass moral judgement but because at a psychological level these behaviours are also seen to involve a distortion of constructive sexual intimacy. For Freud, perversions were an aberration from the "normal aim" of sexual intercourse with the "normal object" of a heterosexual partner (Freud, 1905); Stoller (1975) emphasized the use of sexuality as a vehicle for the expression of hatred rather than love; Limentani (1989) was concerned with the turning away from fundamental psychological "truths" in perversions, such as the truth of generational, gender or species differences (see Wood (2006a) for a fuller discussion of these issues). Psychoanalytic perspectives vary, but what contemporary perspectives all have in common is the notion that, in the perversions, sexualization is used as a means of defending against, managing or masking the anxieties or destructiveness aroused by intimacy, or the "unbearable truths" with which one is confronted through intimacy. In this respect a sexual perversion represents a turning aside, a distortion from proper use or a corruption of intimacy.

In the realm of virtual sex, I think that the addiction model can be used to defend against the "perverse" aspects of these behaviours in this psychoanalytic sense. Specifically an addiction model may protect us from awareness of the predominance of sadism, the use of sexualization as a defence against intolerable affects and the powerful symbolism of the specific scenario on which the individual becomes fixated. All of these—the sadism, the sexualization and the symbolism—may be a source of intense guilt and shame to the individual. The drive to defend against them is powerful and understandable.

The ideas in this chapter are grounded in clinical experience with patients struggling with these issues and are informed by discussion of these issues at the Portman Clinic and elsewhere. The views proposed here are all founded on clinical observation and evidence, but to protect confidentiality no clinical material has been reported directly. Clinical vignettes are fictionalized and therefore serve as illustrations rather than evidence.

There are examples in the literature of people for whom the use of the internet for sexual means is innocuous, sometimes comforting or educational and sometimes potentially very constructive (see for example Tepper and Owens, 2002). In contrast, people attending the Portman Clinic for assessment and treatment all have serious difficulties in the sexual and interpersonal domains and their compulsive use of virtual sex has always seemed to be a symptom, if not a factor compounding these difficulties. The approach that I have taken here assumes that the compulsive use of virtual sex is a problem for the patient.

Different types of users

Initial studies suggest that there may be gender differences in preferred online activities. Men seem to be more likely to engage in solitary activities (viewing and distributing pornography, reading written material) and women are more likely to engage in interactive activity (Ferree, 2003) such as exchanging e-mail, participation in chat rooms and engagement in cybersex (communicating online while masturbating). However, there are women who access pornography, and women are disproportionately represented amongst those who progress beyond recreational use to compulsive or "addictive" use (Cooper, Delmonico, & Burg, 2000). It has also been observed that women are much more likely than men to attempt to have real-life meetings with online sexual partners, with attendant risks.

Carnes, Delmonico and Griffin (2001) have developed a useful typology for distinguishing between different types of users. They refer to "appropriate recreational users", who report no adverse consequences, and "inappropriate recreational users", who are not compulsive users but use sexual information gathered from the internet at inappropriate times or share it with inappropriate people, like colleagues at work. What they call the "predisposed" group already have indicators of problematic sexual behaviour, which seem to be fuelled by the internet. "Lifelong sexual compulsives" have existing problems and may use the internet as an extension of this behaviour as a way to avoid more risky forms of acting out, or to heighten arousal and add new risks to already problematic behaviours. Most interesting from a psychoanalytic point of view is the final group, known as the "discovery group", who reputedly have no prior inappropriate sexual fantasies or behaviours, but for whom the internet serves as a trigger for problematic usage. How should we think about this group? Is it possible that the internet can create disturbed sexual preoccupations where none existed previously? This issue will be discussed below.

From a psychoanalytic point of view, there may be other clinical distinctions to be made between different kinds of problem users. Clinical discussions generate examples of people for whom collecting, sorting and categorizing pornographic images seems paramount, and for whom sexual arousal or masturbation appears to play a minor role. The reasons why pornographic images should be chosen for this purpose may vary, but when coupled with impaired social relating the behaviour may be a feature of Asperger's Syndrome or obsessional-type difficulties. In other people, the imagery or scenario sought out may seem extreme or very severely regressed, involving anatomically almost-impossible acts, or very young infants for example. When coupled with other evidence of a poor reality sense, there may be an impression of an underlying psychotic process, at least in the psychoanalytic, if not in the psychiatric sense. In other people the behaviours seem to be used as an anti-depressant, appearing to offer an escape from a feared state of emptiness and depression. This list is not exhaustive but demonstrates that the compulsive use of virtual sex may be thought of as a symptom, with variable phenomenology and aetiology. There may nevertheless be common features to the function that it serves within the psyche.

Characteristics of the literature

The literature on virtual sex has certain distinct characteristics, which may reflect something about the nature of this as a phenomenon. From a psychoanalytic point of view some of the literature appears to convey a manic excitement.

The global scale of the internet seems to invite expressions of awe. Cooper and Griffin-Shelley (2002) assert that "A new sexual revolution has begun . . .". They assert that the internet has the power to "turbocharge, that is, accelerate and intensify" online sexual activity. Internet pornography is often said to be "the crack cocaine of pornography" (Turpin, 2006; Schneider, 2000), an expression which Griffin-Shelley (2003) attributes to Corley & Corley (1994). Also commonly found in the literature is an expression coined by Cooper (1997), the "triple-A engine", to describe the characteristics of (easy) access, affordability and (apparent) anonymity which lend the internet particular appeal as a vehicle for sexual exploration and expression.

The second distinguishing characteristic of the literature is the huge sample sizes which can be obtained from posting questionnaires on websites. Sample sizes of more than 9,000 (Cooper, Scherer, Boies, & Gordon, 1999), 17,000 (Greenfield, 1999), even 25,000 (Young, 1998) respondents to self-report internet questionnaires are not uncommon. The internet deflects attention away from the single case, and yet in the psychoanalytic tradition it is the single case study which has underpinned theoretical and technical developments and which reveals the subtleties of meaning.

The third conspicuous phenomenon is the creation of a new language, the language of "cybersex", "cyberpsychology", "virtual sex addiction", "cyber stalking", "cyberspace" and "OSA (online sexual activity)". There is even a journal called "CyberPsychology and Behaviour". RL (real life) and f2f (face-to-face) also warrant abbreviations, as if they are just other domains to be visited in a virtual world. The language of cyberspace seems intended to define this phenomenon as scientific, potent and on a vast scale. In "space" the person is weightless, free from the constraints of relationships and the vulnerability bestowed by our ties and our limitations. I would suggest that the language of cyberspace is concerned with a phallic omnipotence.

Within the addiction model it is as though the omnipotence associated with the internet becomes projected into the pornography, which is then seen as an irresistible drug. Greenfield and Orzak (2002), for example, describe how the intoxicating mix of sexual stimulation and the "potent nature of the Internet medium" lead to a situation where a cycle of arousal and compulsion "almost ... spontaneously ignites" (p. 135).

We can credit Rado (1933), an early psychoanalyst, with recognizing the fallacy that an individual is helpless in the face of a potent drug:

> The psychoanalytic study of the problem of addiction begins at this point. It begins with the recognition of the fact that not the toxic agent, but the impulse to use it, makes an addict of a given individual ... The drug addictions are seen to be artificially induced illnesses; they can exist because drugs exist; and they are brought into being for psychic reasons.
>
> [p. 53 in 1997 edition]

Rado points out that the ancient Greeks used the same word to mean "drug" and "magical substance". One of the problems of the addiction model is that we can start to think of the internet and internet sex as though it had an almost magical power. While it is very useful to consider what aspects of internet pornography make it seem so seductive, we know that it is not "irresistible", and it certainly is not magic. The question we need to ask is, what does it offer, not only to the conscious mind, but also to the unconscious, which for some individuals makes it so compelling? And what is it about them that makes them vulnerable to this?

These issues will be explored by considering some similarities between addictions and perversions, and some points of difference.

Similarities between addictions and perversions

The manic high

A feature common to addictions and perversions is the manic high or the elation. Physiologically this may be induced by the chemical effects of a drug, or the pleasure of orgasm through masturbation. Rado (1933) notes that it is only when this physiological high is given meaning by the ego that it yields a subjective sense of elation or omnipotence.

The internet is indeed a technological advance with enormous scope and power. From a psychoanalytic point of view, those very qualities of the internet which render it powerful also bestow a potential for manic excitement and omnipotence. With the smallest gesture, the click of the mouse, the individual can control what happens, the part that they wish to play, and exactly when it should end. The individual can pursue sexual fantasies without any reliance on another person. In the use of pornography there is no unpredictable other who might accept or reject, cherish or criticize them. With both pornography and chat rooms the person can avoid the exposure entailed in intimacy with a partner: exposure of the physical body and aspects of themselves about which they feel ashamed or vulnerable.

Segal (1975) notes that when manic defences are employed, feelings of dependency and vulnerability are replaced by "a triad of feelings—control, triumph and contempt" (Segal, 1975, p. 83). She suggests that: "Control is a way of denying dependence yet compelling the object to fulfil the need for dependence since an object that is wholly controlled is, up to a point, one that can be depended upon." Triumph serves both to devalue the object (and so mitigate any potential feelings of envy), and to counter any feelings such as pining or longing. Contempt also devalues the object and an object that is of no value is not worthy of guilt—the object can be treated mercilessly because its fate is of no consequence. All of these processes can be seen in operation in the use of internet sex. In the mind of the person, the object or the other is totally at their mercy; if there is some live interaction, the other can simply be switched off or terminated if they do not comply with what is sought. The other is frequently dehumanized, allowing the person to feel triumph and contempt. The function of the other is to provide the individual with sexual stimulation and gratification, or to serve as a vessel for the projection of fantasies, but there is no requirement to take account of the other's thoughts, feelings or mind.

Manic defences also serve to spare us from an awareness of our own dependency. While the "primary object" on whom our survival depends is usually seen to be the mother, the body is also a primary object on which we depend, which renders us vulnerable, and whose imperfections we have to recognize and live with. In virtual reality, the person is freed from all bodily constraints—a man can become a woman, a child, an Adonis, a fearless stud. The internet cuts the threads of physical embodiment which always tie us to an imperfect (and "depressive") reality.

A further quality of the internet which may fuel omnipotence and manic defences is the vast array of images available. Someone with a very idiosyncratic sexual fantasy might previously have had little hope of finding that exact fantasy realized. Enactment may therefore have always contained an element of disappointment; the individual cannot control or create external reality to exactly match his wishes or fantasies and omnipotence is thwarted. In contrast, the internet allows the individual to scan vast numbers of images, with the likelihood that any unusual fantasy will eventually find quite a close match. This possibility of finding a match between fantasy and external reality may heighten the sense of omnipotence and excitement (Williams, personal communication).

A common theme in the literature is the disowning of responsibility for the images which are viewed. The distancing effects of scale, technology and anonymity enable the individual to distance himself from guilt about the creation of images. Quayle and Taylor (2002) conducted an impressive study involving qualitative analysis of interviews with 13 men convicted of downloading child pornography. They provide some stark evidence that for some, child pornography became "collectibles", likened by interviewees to baseball cards, stamps, or works of art to be collected, categorized and traded. Respondents would emphasize the importance of collecting complete series, and sorting and categorizing pictures. This was invariably associated with an absence of any reference to the fact that what was being collected was child pornography. Indeed, "Depersonalising of the pictures was seen most strongly when reference was made to the pictures as trophies" (p. 13). In this description, Segal's trio of contempt, control and triumph are once again evident. Manic defences are not simply allowed or endorsed, but seem to be actively fuelled by qualities of the internet.

Even when the internet is used to enact masochistic fantasies in which the individual is debased or made to suffer, that person is secretly in control, dictating the preferred scenario and terminating it when they have had enough. Thus, in the private world of the relationship with the computer, the individual may have the illusion that he or she is supremely powerful and invulnerable, or if this is projected, there may be masochistic gratification in believing that he or she is at the mercy of a supremely powerful other.

Escalation of the "dosage"

Drug use and compulsive use of virtual sex have in common that the elation, the manic high, is ephemeral. It does not effect an enduring state in the psyche. The person has to keep repeating the act to get the high.

Rado suggests that,

> At the height of the elation, interest in reality disappears, and with it any respect for reality.
>
> [p. 57 1997 edition]

As the effects of the drug wear off, the person experiences not just a chemical come-down, but a harsh emotional reawakening.

> The elation had augmented the ego to gigantic dimensions and had almost eliminated reality; now just the reverse state appears,

> sharpened by contrast. The ego is shrunken, and reality appears exaggerated in its dimensions.
>
> [p. 57 ibid]

The addict has a familiar solution to this depressing confrontation with reality: the craving for elation. Rado notes the diminishing returns derived from the state of elation. Progressively more of the drug is needed to effect the required state. He suggests that this effect may be in part physiological and in part psychological.

This is very similar to the pattern we see with compulsive use of virtual sex. It may be due to the guilt induced by the manic flight, the guilt induced by the contempt for the object or the guilt about the sadism expressed, but, once the pleasure of orgasm has worn off, the feeling of depression returns, often amplified. Increasingly desperate attempts to escape the depression may then lead to a search for more extreme material which is seen as more forbidden, more dangerous, and hence, for some, more exciting and more intoxicating. The internet affords the possibility that, when satiation renders the image less exciting or the need to surmount depression is intensified, more extreme versions can be found to heighten arousal. For some people this escalation leads to a search for imagery incorporating increasing levels of violence or increasingly young subjects.

The illusion of an object relationship: a narcissistic relation to a projected internal object

The third striking similarity between drug use and compulsive use of pornography is that there is an illusion of an object relationship, when what is enacted is frequently a narcissistic relation to a projected internal object. The drug user may apparently have a partner, but sexual interest typically wanes, and the partner often becomes more like a business partner, an associate in the business of procuring and funding the drugs. The relationship which is all-consuming is the relationship to the drug, the drug which can be omnipotently controlled and through which the person may enact the incorporation of an idealized object, or an excitingly cruel and dangerous object (see Rosenfeld, 1960).

In the use of virtual sex, the "other" with whom the individual imagines they are engaged, whether it is a person in a static image or a respondent in a chat-room, will only be tolerated while they comply with the scenario that is being sought. Even in chat-rooms where there is a semblance of a relationship, what is engaged with is not an other who embodies difference, nor a transitional space where an individual may safely play with the fantasy of an other (Winnicott, 1951; Gabbard, 2001), but an other who must have fixed characteristics which coincide exactly with the "script" which is sought. The "other" then has no independent existence, but becomes a vessel for the projection of fantasy. The relationship is not one of mutuality, but of narcissistic engagement with a projected internal object.

Mr C sought out imagery in which the participants had to look awkward, unkempt or coarse, so that he could despise and triumph over them in his mind. Mr D, compulsively using chat-rooms where there is an appearance of an other, described himself as "hooking fish". As soon as the other person was seduced by his description of himself and interested in him, he broke off contact with them. The "fish" which he "hooked" were like trophies or junk food—something briefly gratifying but disposable, but far removed from a genuine, sustaining exchange with an other that might have ultimately been nourishing, but which for him was fraught with anxiety.

Differences between compulsive use of virtual sex and drug addiction

The creation of a compelling scenario

A striking feature of virtual sex is the creation of a scenario which is loaded with meaning, a "compelling scenario" (Wood, 2006b). While some might consider that rituals around drug and alcohol use also have this quality, it is not generally a focus of the clinical treatment of these conditions.

In Freud's (with Breuer, 1895) view, "symptoms" are often "overdetermined". In the course of analysis we discover that there is not a single cause, but multiple experiences that seem to have led to this point; one of these experiences alone would probably not have been sufficient to produce or sustain the symptom.

Psychoanalytic exploration often reveals that the particular pornographic scenario upon which an individual becomes fixated has multiple meanings in terms of the person's history, and may have been "over-determined" in the way Freud describes. What the internet appears to offer is a massive library that allows the person to trawl through vast numbers of images or scenarios at great speed, until they alight upon that particular configuration which is, for them, compelling.

For Mr E the participants must be engaged in superhuman sexual feats, offering a fantasized escape from his own feelings of inadequacy and his shame about his life.

The specific sexual scenario may reflect a constellation of object relationships of longstanding significance for the individual. Mr F first had a fantasy of spying on a girl in the neighbourhood in early adolescence when he was socially isolated and unconfident about his appearance. He imagined following her unobserved and observing her relationships with her friends. This fantasy was associated with a generalized excitement but was not at this stage specifically sexual. Over time, Mr F has told me how, as a child feeling helpless in the face of deprivation and abuse, he imagined himself a glamorous (and deadly) international "spy"; how his emotionally unavailable mother would allow him to glimpse her naked while dressing; how enraged he would feel when brutally exposed to evidence of his mother's numerous sexual relationships; and how he imagined that a PE teacher took pleasure in spying on him. "Spying", for him, is suffused with meaning, but it was only in his late teens that he specifically sought out pornographic materials which had to involve the use of concealed cameras to "spy" on scenes of sexual intimacy between children and adults, to reflect what was, by then, an organized sexual fantasy, and which he now pursues on the internet.

I think the addiction model turns a blind eye to the significance of the compelling scenario in collusion with the patient's desire to deny the meaning that it holds. The compelling scenario, like a symptom, may be thought of as a compromise formation. Freud (1896; 1916–17) observed that symptoms, like dreams, represent both the satisfaction of an unconscious wish, and the disguising of that wish through mechanisms such as condensation and displacement. The eventual form of the symptom is thus a "compromise" between the desire for wish-fulfilment and the requirement to comply with the demands of external reality. In practice the symptom very often both conceals and reveals the underlying impulse; the obsessional patient, for example, may simultaneously be washing away every trace of dirt on their hands, while leaving chaos and mess all around them and evoking frustration and rage in those who struggle to engage with them. The messy, aggressive impulses are both washed away and made evident. In the same way, when there is a fixation on a specific sexual scenario, the underlying impulses may be disguised by the sexual scenario, but the disguise is often very flimsy. The compelling scenario both conceals and reveals. What it conceals and reveals is often the most profound, highly charged and sensitive constellations of internal objects. Mr F, described above, could conveniently describe himself as addicted to scenes of covert voyeurism, and he has talked to me about his addiction, as if that explains it all. And yet if we look beyond the surface of the image there may be an underlying fantasy of incest in which he is the mother's chosen partner; there are indications of an ignored and neglected boy in him who longs to be a figure of interest and fascination, projected into the child in the scene; there is an identification with the sexually abusive "aggressor" who violates the child's innocence, and an identification with the power of the "spy" who knows everything that is happening but is unseen. The scenario re-enacts the situation where he feels tantalized and excluded from others' intimacies, but this time he imagines himself in control, cruelly witnessing another's vulnerability, naïveté and abuse. There may be an investment in turning a blind eye to these issues.

Laufer (1976) proposes that the child enters puberty with a "central masturbation fantasy", which may be largely unconscious, but which is an internalized scenario determined by their primary object relationships. In his view, the content of this fantasy "contains the various regressive satisfactions and the main sexual identifications" (p. 300). Laufer considers that this fantasy is fixed by the resolution of the Oedipus complex, and although the fantasy may take on a new meaning in adolescence as the young person assimilates the significance of mature genitals, "*the content of this central masturbation fantasy does not normally alter during adolescence*" (p. 300, his italics). I would question Laufer's insistence that the central fantasy becomes fixed at such an early age since latency and adolescent experiences seem highly influential, but the "compelling scenario" often seems to encapsulate specific traumatic experiences and key object relationships from childhood and adolescence in the way that Laufer describes.

While some people find, through the internet, an external realization of a conscious sexual fantasy, I have come to believe that it is conceivable that, through the internet, some people discover sexual preferences which they might never have discovered through ordinary experience or conscious sexual fantasy. I think it is a mistake to conclude therefore that the internet can somehow "create" a perverse sexual interest like paedophilia. The internet cannot create something from nothing. However, it does seem able to "fan the flames" of something which might otherwise have remained smouldering within the psyche. It seems to do this by intensifying excitement and offering an organized articulation or realization to something that might, without it, have remained largely as disparate unconscious currents within the psyche. The images on which individuals become fixated may seem "novel" because they have not been consciously recognized before, and because they are at odds with the sexual imagery or opportunities generally available in adult life. However, what we find in therapy is that these images or the object relations which they portray are not "new" but are often very "old", referring back to adolescent, Oedipal or pre-Oedipal attachments to bodily functions, body parts, object relationships or primitive fantasies. What the internet provides is, in effect, an invitation to regress, to revisit early or repressed fantasies or experiences. These mental fragments may be highly charged, and so the sexual scenario that gives them form and expression is experienced as compelling.

Sexualization and sexualization of aggression

The second major difference between drug addiction and perversion is the extent of the sexualization, and specifically the sexualization of aggression in perversion. Drug use undoubtedly gratifies destructive urges, and there may be a perverse pleasure in the attack on the self, the body or the imagined objects who suffer or are punished. However, perversions are distinguished by the fact that destructive wishes are not simply libidinalized or eroticized, but are actually sexualized—woven into a specific and concrete sexual fantasy or act.

Psychoanalytic theorists such as Glasser (1979) and Stoller (1975) have emphasized the way in which perversions allow the sexualization of hatred and aggression, in a way that disguises and appears to "make safe" the aggression. Stoller stresses the aetiological importance of experiences in which the individual is humiliated with regard to their sexuality or gender, thus storing up hatred and a desire for revenge upon the object. Stoller argues that the perverse act—in many of his examples, transvestism—gratifies the desire for revenge. In the cross-dressing ritual the man appears to repeat what has been done to him, denies his masculinity and assumes the identity of a woman, but at the end of the ritual he masturbates and ejaculates, reasserting his masculinity and mentally triumphing over those who have humiliated or denigrated him. This is a re enactment in which history is re-written: through sexualization, the apparent re-enactment of the trauma culminates in his pleasure and triumph.

In his view, the scenario on which the individual becomes fixated, whether it be cross dressing or an obsession with pornography, puts the individual in the superior, vengeful, triumphant position. The other is seen to suffer, and their suffering is a source of satisfaction and pleasure. Thus the original "victim" becomes "victor", "trauma" becomes "triumph" and "passive suffering" becomes "active revenge".

Mr G, who became fixated on sado-masochistic homosexual imagery, tells me how, when he started to look at this material, he was feeling unable to cope with his high-pressure job, was failing in relationships and felt he was falling apart. He identifies the victim in the imagery with himself as a child, physically and emotionally abused and "treated worse than a dog". And yet witnessing another being treated in this way gives him pleasure. The projection on to the victim of all that he could not bear to experience or own, is driven by rage and functions in his mind as an act of aggression; when coupled with sexualization, and elaborated into a specific fantasy, it becomes a source of sadistic pleasure.

For Glasser (1979a) it is the aggression aroused by core complex anxieties which is sexualized and made safe in perversions. He describes how what he calls the core complex arises as a response to frustration in early relationships resulting from separation. In the core complex the response to this frustration is to pursue a search for blissful union with the object, which appears to promise the eradication of deprivation and need, and the total containment of destructive feelings. In those with perverse pathology, Glasser suggests that this primitive urge for union arouses a terror of annihilation—to be completely taken over by another is to lose oneself—and therefore arouses intense feelings of aggression against the object. Yet to destroy the object would be to be left without any hope of gratification, isolated, depressed and abandoned. Mr H described graphically in his first assessment session how he longed for a kind of back-in-the-womb-type experience in which he was completely fused with another. He went on to say how he felt completely pent up, like an atomic reactor about to explode. He made the link that his use of internet pornography was his way of diffusing the charge, essentially the rage, that he felt inside, although he had not made the link that this rage was a response to the regressive and primitive longing for fusion. Internet pornography thus provides him with an apparent solution to core complex anxieties.

In this group of patients for whom virtual sex, in its different forms, has become severely problematic, the virtual sex always seems to function, at least in part, to express sadistic impulses towards the object. Prior to and after breaks in the therapy, Mr J seeks out imagery on the internet in which women are treated sadistically. He has the satisfaction of "leaving" me and our work together, and taking off into his own world of pornography where I cannot contact him. Thus he reverses the situation where he is left by me in the break and takes revenge on me in his mind as Stoller describes. Through the pornography he also sexualizes the aggression and appears to discharge it and make it safe, so that he protects me in the consulting room from the full weight of his angry and vengeful feelings. He also protects himself from acknowledging the pain of separation and the depth of his longings. As Glasser describes, the perversion protects the relationship to the object which the individual fears might otherwise be destroyed by the aggression.

Ambiguity about internal / external reality

One of the particularly interesting aspects of the use of virtual sex is the ambiguity about whether or not this constitutes enactment or fantasy. Is this taking place in external reality? Or in internal reality? Or somewhere in between?

The lawyer, teacher or hospital consultant who stands to lose everything if found guilty of looking at child pornography presumably convinces himself when looking at internet pornography that this is taking place solely in internal reality, in his mind. I am struck by how often, in discussion of this subject with colleagues, someone takes it upon themselves to remind us all that real children are involved in the production of child pornography, as if we could all be carried away by the illusion that this is all in the mind, and so, in effect, without consequence to anyone but the user. Taylor and Quayle's (2003) sobering book about the production and use of child pornography is a valuable reminder of the processes involved. For some patients, the ambiguity about whether it is external or internal, real or fantasy, seems an almost psychotic riddle which they find very disturbing. For others, it may be a source of additional charge or excitement, enhancing a sense of danger or risk. The person may be both excited by and frightened by the thought that they might be caught, or might be unable to stop themselves from enacting what they had witnessed. For some, exploiting the ambiguity about whether what they are doing is virtual or real becomes part of the excitement. As it is not illegal to fantasize or to look, but only to possess images, ever more sophisticated technological means may be employed to delete images, to destroy the "footprint" left on the computer and to leave no trace. In this way the individual may imagine triumphing over external authority (the police, the criminal justice system) by obliterating the evidence that this was enacted in external reality, and creating a pretence that it occurred only in the mind.

The role of the superego

When working with perverse patients, qualities of the superego are often known initially from projections on to the psychotherapist. The therapist may feel themselves to be alternately perceived to be ineffectual, weak and collusive, actively corrupt and seductive, or severely judgmental and punitive. Such projections may have their origins in actual childhood experiences of active seduction and abuse or the failure of parental figures to protect, as well as in early experiences in which the primitive qualities of the superego were fuelled by fantasy and destructiveness (see for example Glasser's (1988) account of the poor integration and hence primitive nature of the superego in paedophilia).

At the simplest level, the internet may appear to invite a disregard for authority because, alone in a room with a computer, the individual imagines that there are no witnesses to their actions. Their awareness of external controls (such as social disapproval or the law), and the self-consciousness associated with this, may be eroded (Young, 2003).

Constraints on an individual's behaviour also derive from internal controls, the functions of conscience, self-observation and ideals of behaviour that we associate with the superego. The internet may be a convenient object for projections of qualities of the superego. Where the internet has become the focus of compulsive sexual activity, the internet is often identified with a corrupt or seductive superego, and the therapist (and sometimes the criminal justice system) are alternately seen to be weak and helpless, or harsh, judgmental and persecutory.

The internet has many of the characteristics of a powerful parent: it knows "everything", it is immediately responsive, it can be summoned at will and it relieves boredom and loneliness. The projection on to it of a parental, and perhaps specifically paternal, authority is thus not remarkable. However, the internet is also a parent who never says "no". Indeed, elaborate systems exist to tempt the user to remain online, to visit additional websites or to scan more extreme imagery. The pornographic imagery, or the expressed sexual preference, appear to bear the stamp of social approval or endorsement, because there are clearly other people who share this fantasy and have posted the image or information on the internet. Chat-rooms, where it is possible to exchange views with others with socially proscribed sexual interests, appear to normalize the specific sexual interest and create a sense that this is representative of a sub-set of society and hence not "deviant", thus allowing the triumph of a corrupt superego over ordinary social mores. The possibility of breaking the law and then deleting all evidence of the crime may further fuel the sense that the internet works in the service of a corrupt authority, and lends itself to acts of triumph over a watchful conscience.

Everyone has within them a sexually curious child, the Oedipal child who wonders what goes on behind the door of the parental bedroom. It is as if the internet plays on people's sexual curiosity, symbolically beckoning the "child" into the parental bedroom with the promise of satisfying their sexual curiosity. Just as the reality of exposure to the primal scene may be profoundly disturbing to a child, so many people report seeing imagery on the internet to which they subsequently wish they had not been exposed.

There is anecdotal evidence that people with sexual addiction have commonly had early exposure to pornography, and it is striking how frequently patients refer to the discovery in early adolescence of pornography belonging to the father or a male relative. In these situations it is as though the father no longer embodies prohibition, the "no" of the Oedipal father, but is seen to be unable to contain his own polymorphous sexual interests, his own sadism or masochism, and his own voyeurism. The developing superego of the boy may bear the imprint of his identification with a corrupt or perverse paternal object.

For those who develop a compulsive interest in internet pornography, the breaching of social boundaries and taboos may not be just an unfortunate side-effect of their pursuit of specific sexual preferences, but a vital part of the behaviour. There is pleasure in transgression, in breaking social norms and taboos.

The damage to the superego is unlikely to occur in a single trauma and there may be other developmental factors contributing to this fragility or breaching of the superego. The impact of a mother who "turns a blind eye" and is seen to be complicit in the father's practices may also be considerable. But in some vulnerable patients, the corrupt internet "parent" who seems to invite exploration without restraint may find resonance with a part of them that derives pleasure from breaching boundaries and taboos.

Summary

I have come to believe that there are aspects of the internet which render the pursuit of virtual sex particularly "addictive" in a functional sense. The access to powerful and exciting technology, the possibility of a fit between a sexual fantasy and external reality, the degree of control afforded to the individual and the absence of any other with vitality and a will of their own, the promised gratification of sexual curiosity, sealed by the excitement of sexual orgasm—all these can fuel omnipotence, and can seem very intoxicating. However, to see compulsive use of virtual sex as "just" an addiction is at best misleading, and at worst, may collude with a defensive denial of the perverse aspects of the behaviour. The compulsive use of virtual sex has all the hallmarks of a perversion: it is a fixed, repetitive, often ritualized sexual behaviour, in which sexualization is used as a defence against profound disturbances in object relations and the relationship to reality. The behaviours are frequently underpinned by narcissistic disturbances, profound feelings of depression, and destructive wishes and annihilatory anxieties in relation to the object. A psychoanalytic approach to treatment offers the possibility of unravelling the highly-charged and sensitive constellation of fantasy, object relations and anxieties underpinning the behaviour, thereby leading to a reduction in the charge or compulsion to enact.

CHAPTER TEN

Trans-sexuality

A case of the "Emperor's new clothes"

Az Hakeem

There was once a rather narcissistic Emperor whose only concerns were those of appearance. His love of fine clothes was known throughout his Kingdom and before long a couple of entrepreneurial young men appeared at the palace with a scheme in mind. They presented themselves as master craftsmen, tailors who had invented an extraordinary method of weaving gold thread into a fine cloth which was so fine as to be almost invisible. In fact, they suggested that to anyone who was too stupid or incompetent to appreciate its fine quality, it would indeed appear to be invisible.

The Emperor duly arranged for no expense to be spared and the two craftsmen applied for much gold thread, in order for a new set of clothes to be made for the Emperor. On supposed completion of this piece of miracle tailoring, the Prime Minister was sent to inspect the new clothes. On seeing the new garment the Prime Minister could see nothing, but on fear of being seen as stupid or incompetent and being discharged from his office, he went against his better judgement and declared it to be a most marvellous fabric.

Finally, the Emperor was presented with his new clothes by the two young men. He too could see nothing but he too was frightened of being seen as stupid and incompetent—so instead he pretended he could see the clothes and praised the quality of work and colours of the material. Seeing that their scheme was working, the two young men informed the Emperor that he would have to take off his clothes in order to try on his new suit. Although internally embarrassed the Emperor did this, and was reassured by those around him who seemed to be showing signs of approval of the fine fabric and craftsmanship, but they too were scared of being seen as stupid or incompetent fools.

The Prime Minister informed the Emperor that word had spread throughout the Kingdom of his fine new suit and that the public wished to see the Emperor in his amazing new clothes. The narcissistic Emperor granted the people this privilege and arranged for a ceremonial procession to take place. The crowds along the procession applauded, cheered and unanimously praised the fine fabric, the colours, and the craftsmanship, declaring what a beautiful suit the Emperor wore—although none of them could see any fabric, they all wished to conceal their disappointment that they too were incompetent and stupid for not being able to see the clothes.

Eventually, a small boy went up to the carriage. This boy had no important status to preserve, and could only see things as his eyes showed him, "The Emperor is naked!", he declared. The boy's father reprimanded him and tried to silence him, calling him a foolish boy. However, the crowd who had heard the boy's comment started to repeat what they had heard. "The boy is right, the Emperor is naked, it's true!" The Emperor realised the people were right and was filled with unhappiness and regret. However, he was a proud man and did not want to admit that he had made a mistake, and decided to continue the procession under the illusion that anyone who could not see his clothes was either stupid or incompetent. He remained standing on his carriage, whilst behind him a page held his imaginary mantle. (Andersen, 1857)

Historical aspects

Trans-sexuality is generally understood to be a state in which an individual who is biologically and unambiguously a member of one sex holds the strong belief that he or she is in fact a member of the opposite sex. It is not a new condition and has a long history spanning as far back as the time of the Assyrian King Sardanapalus, around 800 BC, who was reported to have been slain due to the outrage he caused dressing in female clothing, wearing make-up and adopting a female identity. More recently, the first clearly documented cases of gender reassignment surgery were those of Lili Elbe in Dresden 1930, and Christine Jorgensen in Copenhagen 1951 (Sorenson & Hertoft, 1980). The term "trans-sexual" began entering into popular usage in the early 1960s around the time that dominant names in the field of gender dysphoria such as Robert Stoller (Stoller, 1968; 1975), John Money and Franke Erhardt (1972) and others started investigating the condition. Around half-a-century after the conception of this apparent third gender, trans-sexuality continues to be a cause of much controversy. Despite this controversy there appears to be very little debate about our understanding of the condition that causes concern to myself as having an interest in this field.

Psychiatric approaches to trans-sexuality

A recent article published in the *Psychiatric Bulletin* proposed to outline the services seen to be providing "appropriate treatment for trans-sexual patients" (Jurgen *et al.*, 2002). The authors of the article refer to the standards of care for trans-sexuals that are internationally recognized and laid down by the Harry Benjamin International Gender Dysphoria Association (HBIGDA) (2002). The HBIGDA is an international body of professionals who have produced definitive guidelines to which clinicians working with trans-sexual patients are advised to adhere. The authors of the recent article list the management of the trans-sexual patient as including diagnostic assessment, supportive psychotherapy, the "real life experience", hormonal therapy and surgery. In a way rather similar to the various interpretations of religious text by differing religious organizations, it seems that the authors of this article have their own interpretation and understanding of what the treatment for trans-sexuals is. In their article there are many assumptions made which seem to be based on presumption rather than clinical experience. Such ideas included the presumption that conventional interpretative psychotherapy is not indicated and that the mainstay of appropriate treatment for trans-sexuals is physically or surgically orientated, including genital re-construction, hysterectomy, mastectomy or breast enlargement and cricothyroid surgery in men. With such ideas coming from the minds of psychiatrists, it seems very difficult to attempt to understand the mind of a trans-sexual.

A psychoanalytic approach to trans-sexuality

The rather concrete approach by many psychiatrists voiced by the authors of the article mentioned above is in contrast to the more psychoanalytically informed understanding of psychoanalysts and psychoanalytic psychotherapists and psychiatrists, including myself. There is a long tradition of attempting to understand the trans-sexual condition at the Portman Clinic which was pioneered by the eminent psychiatrist and psychoanalyst, Dr Adam Limentani, and his work with such patients at the Portman Clinic in the early 1970s. He saw patients in an analytic setting over several years and formulated an understanding of these patients which was later to appear in his chapter on the condition in his collected works, *Between Freud and Klein: The Psychoanalytic Quest for Knowledge and Truth* (1989). Limentani's interest in this group of patients encouraged others at the Clinic, and within the field, to similarly develop an enthusiasm for treating these patients in a psychoanalytically informed manner in an attempt to understand them and to help them understand themselves. In more recent years, in addition to such patients being treated over long periods of time for individual psychoanalytic psychotherapy, there has also been a psychotherapy group at the Portman Clinic for post-operative trans-sexual patients who were referred in a state of despair and mourning as a result of a course of action they had been allowed to progress through, and also a psychotherapy group which was started nine years ago for preoperative trans-sexual patients and those with gender dysphoria.

If the definition of a delusion is that of being a firmly held, unshakeable false-belief then surely the conviction that one is what one is not is also understood as a delusional disorder. Some years ago, whilst on call as a Senior House Officer in Psychiatry, I was asked to see a woman who had been brought in to the unit and who was crawling around the floor naked, making cat-like noises. The woman, at that point in time, believed that she was a cat. The management of this patient that I thought appropriate was not to collude with her delusional belief and convince myself that she was a cat, but instead to try and understand her condition as being an encapsulated psychosis. To suggest that the core belief defining an individual as a trans-sexual—the belief that one is the gender that one is not—be understood as an encapsulated mono-delusional belief is surprisingly controversial. The very nature of the delusion being encapsulated means that such individuals are not "psychotic" in the same way as, for example, a person with active schizophrenia or another disintegrative condition and explains why such individuals are able to function as perfectly able and capable human beings who do not appear to be affected in any other way than their apparent convictions over their gender. It seems very hard for psychiatrists to challenge the fundamental core belief of the trans-sexual and examine with them what actually it is to be the opposite sex or indeed, more importantly, what it is to be any sex, without falling into the trap of personally or socially constructed actual or mythical gender stereotypes.

Although the example of the patient who thought she was a cat can be seen as anecdotal, we must ask ourselves why we really separate such individuals with false beliefs relating to their gender from individuals who hold other false beliefs such as the person with "anoptophilia" who believes they are a partial person trapped in a complete person's body and pursue surgery in order to remove a fully functioning limb or body part which they believe they should never have owned. It is interesting that the medical profession has chosen to split off trans-sexual patients with a gender related mono-delusional belief from such other patients. With surgery allowing us to be increasingly creative, we perhaps believe that we can become the "ultimate creator" which satisfies a need to take up the role of superhero or magician who can eradicate the problems of our patients with some magical manoeuvre. Perhaps this is not too dissimilar to the entrepreneurial craftsmen in the tale of the Emperor. The hope is that we will be held in high esteem by our patients for providing them with what they apparently wanted. The danger is that we may actually become more like Dr Frankenstein (Shelley, 1818).

It seems strange that as psychiatrists we attempt to address an internal psychological conflict with an exterior surgical solution almost as if we were performing neurosurgery by operating on a person's genitalia. It is also of concern that psychoanalytic psychotherapy is presumed either unsuccessful or perhaps too expensive even as a treatment option for these patients, and I wonder whether it is also presumed to be too politically incorrect even to question the false-belief systems of these individuals. It seems that psychotherapists and psychoanalytically informed psychiatrists represent the little boy in the story of the Emperor's new clothes and stand alone whilst the kingdom around them wants to be seen to be colluding with an overwhelming false belief.

Long-term, exploratory work with trans-sexual patients either in individual or group psychotherapy has brought new insights to the understanding of how such a condition may arise in individuals. The trans-sexual condition can be thought of as a "solution" to an internal conflict that would otherwise be unbearable and intolerable, perhaps almost to the point of a psychotic breakdown and a more generalized disintegration of the mental state. It was Dr Edward Glover, one of the founding psychiatrists of the Portman Clinic, who observed that sometimes a perversion is a defence against psychosis (1933). Whilst I am not suggesting that the trans-sexual solution is necessarily a perversion in this sense of the word, I do believe that it has a number of functions of a defensive kind, as I have seen in a number of my patients.

Patient C describes a life-long state of depersonalization and feels that she has never had an identity of her own including that of gender or sexuality. She believes that if she were to become a man by having a "sex change" then she could become a "real" person. Patient C is an example of an individual for whom trans-sexuality seems to be a defence against a more generalized psychotic breakdown.

Patient A, a retired ex-marine in his 50s, previously married and a father, attempted to become a young woman in her mid-thirties initially by cross-dressing and later by hormonal and surgical intervention. Like many trans-sexuals, for Patient A his trans-sexuality seemed to be a defence against the ageing process and the switch to another gender would enable a new lease of life, either physically or psychologically for that individual.

Patient F had spent most of his life feeling unhappy and alone. His sense of isolation and depression was worsened since his migration to this country where after thirty years he still felt close to no-one. He had felt for most of his life that if only he had been born a woman he would be much happier. For Patient F, like many patients, trans-sexuality functions as a hope against an overwhelming depression.

Patient B in his early 30s realizes he is male. However Mr B, who had a very religious upbringing, detests the idea of homosexuality and believes that in order to have a relationship with a man he would have to become a woman. As a population sub-group there is a significant degree of veiled intolerance towards homosexuality and hostility towards women amongst trans-sexuals. Patients in my group have described their abhorrence of homosexuality and how as men they would need to become women to enable them to have the sexual relations they desire with other men as they "could not possibly be gay". Other patients have held the belief that by removing their male genitalia, creating an artificial vaginal space and acquiring breasts, they would become women. In the trans-sexual, the gender of the chosen sexual object may not come into question but instead it is their very own gender that is being disputed. Surely such a notion of what it is to be a woman is not too far from that proposed by the misogynist.

The trans-sexual must also be differentiated from the transvestite, who does not have a conviction that he should be a woman but instead gains satisfaction by going inside his mother's skin (the female clothing) and then takes it off again. This model of understanding the transvestite is one described by Dr Mervin Glasser, a former psychiatrist at the Portman Clinic, in his paper *Analysis of a Transvestite* (1979). The ability to engage in such temporary "residencies" within the mother can become a source of pleasure and for some even develop into a sexual fetish. This is in contrast to the male trans-sexual who wishes to be female and wants no such temporary residency within his mother. For such trans-sexuals it is not a case of excitement or sexual fetish, but for them one possible understanding is that if they cannot *have* their mother then they will attempt to be their mother, as described by Coates and Person (1985). They are not interested in renting, but buying, and are seeking permanent residence in the body of the mother.

Of course there is no simple or straightforward explanation for the condition, as indeed there does not seem to be for the other conditions we treat in psychiatry. Many of the trans-sexual patients seen at the Portman Clinic give histories of great adversity and confusion spanning most of their life, many having been born as replacement children following previous babies who have been lost due to miscarriage or early childhood death and who have been of the opposite gender. Other patients were made more overtly aware that their parents would have preferred a child of the opposite sex, being dressed in clothes usually associated with the opposite gender or being given gender non-specific names and treated asexually throughout their upbringing. Patient J was brought up in a household of aunts and a grandmother who dressed him as a girl in handmade smocks in which they dressed his five sisters also. He felt no different from his sisters and was horrified when at puberty he started to develop as a man.

Other patients have described particular traumas associated with one of their parents. Patient D resents his father as he blames him for his mother's death. D had discovered the dead body of his mother after she committed suicide when D was aged 10. Perhaps in this individual the trans-sexual solution is both an attack on the father and also an attempt at keeping his mother alive.

Explanations for the condition that ignore the internal world and the development of the minds of these patients and instead try to explain it in a purely biological way, seem to be missing the point. Attempts to provide one single, simple biological determinant or explanation, which no study has ever successfully been able to achieve, seem to be an attempt to reduce something very complex into something as far too simple and fail to see beyond the presenting symptom itself. Such a flight away from mindfulness may be a reflection of how difficult it is to try and think about the disturbance created in the trans-sexual mind.

Gender reassignment

The term "gender reassignment surgery" or "sex change operation" is a misnomer. Of course, one cannot actually change gender. Georges Burou, the famous surgeon who performed such operations in Casablanca, is quoted as saying "I do not change men into women. I transform male genitals into genitals which have a female aspect. All the rest is in the patient's mind" (1974). Although surgery seems to have become the presumed form of "appropriate treatment" for this population, there seems to be scant, if any, evidence-based research or follow-up studies to back this up as an appropriate form of treatment. This leads to the question as to why no follow-up studies of any significant length are performed for this population post-operation. The response which has been given to me by clinicians involved is that once they have had an operation these patients no longer want to be medicalized and treated as patients and want to be free to live their own lives.

The post-operative trans-sexual

Whilst such surgery may offer help to some patients and there is no doubt that some are more comfortable in themselves, what about the unfortunate patients for whom surgery does not provide a resolution to their serious internal conflict? For eight years Dr Elif Gurisik ran a once weekly psychotherapy group for post-operative trans-sexuals at the Portman Clinic. Prior to this she had spent a number of years treating similar patients with individual psychoanalytic psychotherapy. These individuals who had been referred to the clinic were presenting with degrees of dissatisfaction or unhappiness following their operation. Many of them felt a great deal of anger and resentment for being allowed to undergo a process which they now regarded as leaving them mutilated and neither male nor female. The group was considered very successful for these individuals and although in real terms nothing could be done on a physical basis for them, many reported that one of the functions of the group was to prevent them from committing suicide. Unfortunately, no such group for postoperative trans-sexuals exists outside the clinic. The Portman Clinic continues to receive a steady flow of referrals of patient who had "sex changes" and are now in a state of despair and confusion and are seeking therapeutic help. To my knowledge there is no such psychological breakdown service provided by the very centres which provide the mechanical transformations for these individuals. It will perhaps be interesting to perform lifelong follow-up studies to see how many of these patients actually do become more fulfilled by surgical manoeuvres as well as to determine the incidents of depression and the rates of suicide in this post-operative population.

Group psychotherapy for the pre-operative transsexual and gender dysphoric patient

The other group for trans-sexual patients at the clinic is the group for individuals who have not had gender reassignment surgery. These patients may regard themselves as trans-sexual, trans-gendered or gender-dysphoric. This therapy group was started by Dr Estela Welldon and has been run by me for the past six years. This slow-open group is indeed a very interesting challenge. Since the group started there have been a number of noticeable shifts within the group of patients. When the patients enter the group there is often a predominance of rather rigid ways of thinking concretely, especially about their gender, with much identification with very conservative gender role behaviour and stereotyped attributes. In the group their ideas and beliefs are able to be examined and challenged, not only by the therapist but also by each other. This is one way in which group psychotherapy for this population has an advantage over individual psychotherapy, in my opinion. What is noticeable is that the focus on the external world gradually shifts to focusing more on their own internal world and through working in the group they foster an ability to be able to question ideas which they have previously held with a firm conviction for a considerable, if not life-long, period, which become more malleable and are able to be questioned. One group member told another in a session, "I completely agree with everything you've just said, but listening to you saying it makes it seem completely mad!"

The relationship between forensic psychotherapy and the trans-sexual

Recently when giving talks introducing the concept of forensic psychotherapy and mentioning group therapy for trans-sexual patients, I have been asked why I believe the therapy of these patients comes under the auspices of forensic psychotherapy. It is at this point that

I wish to refer you back again to the story of the Emperor's new clothes. The link between the story and the issue of the trans-sexual is the concept of fraud and deception which, in my opinion, is evident in this phenomenon in a number of ways. To refer to Dr Welldon, "deception can indeed be a very artistic endeavour" (2001) and in the trans-sexual it is the artistry with which we have found ourselves helping them, which attempts to take it away from reality and the painful internal conflict. In a recent session of my group one member had commented how he had spent some time with a friend of his who was undergoing a "sex change" and how, despite considering himself a trans-sexual, he described a state of intense discomfort and feeling rather disturbed by being in the presence of his friend. He felt that he could not relate to him as either a male or female but that he has become a "non-gendered person". This was followed by another member recounting to the group the recent experience of being in a restaurant where an individual who was clearly a male to female trans-sexual had entered the restaurant and sat at a table. He described how this individual's trans-gendered status was clear to everyone but how nobody "battered an eyelid". He used this as an example of how widely accepted trans-sexuals are in our current society. This is an illustration of how for some trans-sexual patients appearances really do seem to be everything. Although people may not only see through the deceptive facade and experience a state of disturbance or discomfort, the important thing seems to be *whether or not they are seen to be* experiencing any disturbance or *seen to have* realized that it is a facade. Thus if people are seen to accept them for who they are attempting to be, then that was all that mattered, and even if the reality and the internal belief of these people was contrary to this, this did not matter. This fear of confrontation is almost a "folie à deux".

This takes us back again to the story of the Emperor, where it was the young boy who had the freedom to express his honest feelings who was able to be true to himself and not collude with the madness and deception he found all around him. It is interesting that one of my patients has reported that an indicator of how convincing he is as a woman, or how successful the deception is, is to walk down the street in public around the time that schools are closing. The very politically incorrect honesty mixed with the unfortunate cruelty of children allow this individual to gauge whether he is successful in his endeavours of deceit and control of others when the level of remarks passed by children will be few. In contrast, if his deception is unsuccessful this will be manifest in much taunting and humiliation. It seems that in our profession it is only the psychoanalytical psychotherapist or the similarly informed psychiatrist (and only the more vocal, braver ones at that) who take on the role of the boy in the story and are able to represent the voice of reality rather than the voice of the perceived majority who are seen to collude with the fantasy and deception.

Legislative changes

A recent ruling in the European Court of Human Rights resulted in the decision that a postoperative male to female trans-sexual had the right to marry a biological male (2002). In response to this, I and a number of other clinicians wrote a letter which appeared in the national press stating our views on the condition and how we felt that such a decision by the European Court of Human Rights was a victory for fantasy over reality and that our concerns were that the problems and conflicts within the trans-sexually conflicted individual may not be wholly solved by either surgical or legal manoeuvres (Berkowitz *et al.*, 2002). The response to the letter from trans-sexual individuals and other groups was extensive and we received numerous irate and inflamed letters (Hamilton, 2002). Of interest was that the complaints being made were not due to the specifics of the content of our letter but more directed by the fact that we dared to air an opinion which was described in one letter as "not the current medically or legally accepted viewpoint". Such phrasing would suggest that the world of medicine is united in embracing the collusion with this widespread deception that a person can actually change their sex and that to voice the opinion that they may think otherwise could be considered illegal.

Of course, neither I nor any of the other clinicians with whom I work are opposed to a trans-sexual being allowed the right to marry but our objections are that they be allowed as *a person of the sex which they are not*. If legislation was to change to allow individuals of the same sex to marry, then this would enable trans-sexuals to marry individuals of either gender without problems. It seems that the recent ruling is a step backwards for the fight for the right of same-sex marriage, an issue which affects homosexuals in this country and to prevent them from having the opportunity of marriage. It seems that rather than change this legislation (although the recent developments in 'civil partnerships' goes some way towards this), the ruling for trans-sexuals implies that it is not acceptable for members of the same sex to marry with the exception that *it is acceptable if one of the sexes can at least have the suitably deceptive appearance of being the other sex.*

A similarly related ongoing battle currently in process is the fight for the trans-sexual to be allowed to change the gender specified on their birth certificate. Again, we are faced with deception. A birth certificate is a record of one's gender at a certain point in time: our birth. Even if in the realms of fantasy an individual was actually able to change sex later in life, this does not change the fact that at birth they were born in the original gender. In the same way as the vehicle licensing document shows details of the car at the point of original registration irrespective of what later mechanical or structural changes are made to the car. To try to change the details on one's birth certificate is a deceptive attempt to breach the concept of time and history retrospectively and can be understood as an act of magical undoing. It seems that in the attempt to retain political correctness and to appease a vociferous population, the correct understanding of what a birth certificate represents is lost and it takes the meaning of a document certifying current gender identity.

A further illustration of the deception would be the possibility arising in the event of both the aforementioned pieces of legislation. They could result in a man marrying what he presumed to be a woman who had a female passport, a birth certificate declaring him to be female at time of birth, who is taken to be female and an individual whom he believed he could marry and who could be the mother of his children but in reality his wife actually being a man.

The future

A few years ago the Royal Society of Medicine organized a one-day conference devoted to the future planning of treatment resources for trans-sexual patients (2002). During this day there was a distinct scarcity of any attempts at psychological understanding of these individuals or of helping them to understand themselves or to treat the conflict in any other way other than surgically. Other than the therapeutic group which I run at the Portman Clinic, I know of no other form of psychoanalytically based psychotherapy group or other clinicians in the UK offering a forum for transsexual or gender dysphoric patients to understand themselves. Instead, there seems to be an abundance of interest in achieving a fine tuning of surgical procedures in the hope that this will offer a "long-term solution" to these patients' problems. Our extensive collected experience in working with these patients psychoanalytically at the Portman Clinic and attempting to understand their trans-sexual conflict has proved that there is no simple, unified aetiology for this condition and we feel that a single treatment approach, especially one involving little or no psychological input, is of great concern. At present, the only psychological input to their treatment consists of an initial screening to rule out DSM IV, Axis I type major psychotic conditions (American Psychiatric Association, 2000). This is followed by the psychiatric profession entering into the ultimate collusion with the psychosis manifest in their insistence that these patients dress up and live in their desired gender role for two years, in order to ascertain how successful the deceptive process can be. I sincerely hope that in planning future treatment resources or implementing any treatment frameworks for this population, fundamental and important areas such as the work in which we are currently involved is not overlooked and is considered during planning processes. Our recent letter and undoubtedly this paper as well will provoke a reaction and debate, but this can only be seen as a positive step in the field which has otherwise been focused along a rather narrow trajectory.

CHAPTER ELEVEN

Perverse patients' use of the body—their own and that of others

David Morgan

In this chapter I will briefly describe a number of patients and my clinical experience of them to illustrate how the patient's use of the body or inanimate objects may be understood to be an unconscious attempt to manage or change emotional conflicts through enacting them on the body – their own or someone else's. This might be considered to be a reflection of the patients own early experience of being reacted to at a purely physical level rather than at an emotional or mental level. It is said that some patients – and those displaying violence, perversion and delinquincy would definitely come into this category – do not have a sufficient capacity to use their mind and resort to the use of the body as their only means of expression and communication.

A patient's memory of his early childhood was the rubber mattress that he used to turn to as a child when he felt abandoned by his mother. This can be seen as a defensive retreat to a stable or reliable object over which he could exert power and control. His destructive feelings towards his mother were so great that he had to destroy his knowledge of his need for her and give it to an inanimate substance. In later life this had developed into a full rubber fetish and he would climb into a wetsuit, which acted as an auto erotic substitute at times of intimacy with his wife. This forced her into a subservient position, putting her into the role of accomplice and voyeur to his exhibitionism. Thus he eliminates his own experiences of helplessness at the hands of his early relationships by reversing them and through a process of projective identification puts these feelings into the other, whilst he retains the relationship with the primary object by imbuing a lifeless substance with power, whilst asset stripping his wife. This is a common constellation in the presentation of patients with perversions and/or addictions. Human relationships are asset stripped and subordinated to objects and substances which become idealized, thus ensuring that human attachment with all its inherent dangers of loss, death and dependency can be avoided. Clearly this is often caused by very early failures of attachment but can also be due to excessive destructiveness and envy towards creativity and the capacity for love in others. Inanimate objects are sexualized and the knowledge of the need for love from others is destroyed. Thus aggression and anxiety caused by early fears of disintegration become eroticized and powerful rather than disintegrating into a terrifying descent into psychosis.

If a part of one's own body, clothes and other substances becomes fetishized in this way then the accompanying fantasy is that the source of gratification is in the pursuit of this. The other people involved play a secondary role replicating the earliest experience of attachment where the object may have been felt to be unavailable or preoccupied. A patient I saw who was a young psychiatrist had a fetishistic relationship with cutting her arms, particularly around breaks. She had a post-puerperally depressed mother from birth. Our understanding of her cutting was that it was her way of reversing an unbearable situation with a mother who was unable to contain her daughter's anxiety about survival. Dr T had reversed this unbearable situation by becoming the one who caused anxieties about her own survival in others. This was both a reversal of the dangerous aggression that she feared her mother would not be able to manage by attacking her own body, and also in the early years of therapy with me a method of discovering whether I could bear these complex and frightening emotions around death and mutilation that she threatened me with.

In other fetishists the role of the other is all-important. For instance, a transvestite is often married but like the television personality and her stooge Madge the real woman is triumphed over and turned into a secondary woman. I have been impressed by the number of wives of transvestites who have had hysterectomies at an early age, perhaps the result of murderous attacks on the one aspect of being a woman that cannot yet be replicated.

Heimann (1952) states: "... the essential difference between infantile and mature object relations is that, whereas the adult conceives of the object as existing independently of himself, for the infant it always refers in some way to itself." This description of object relations encompasses introjection in which the object becomes identified with a part of themselves, and hence the infant sucks his thumb and feels himself to be in contact with the breast. This creates fantasies of having incorporated the breast and a feeling that he can produce his own gratification. Thus pathological narcissism is a state of auto-erotic gratification. In the perversions we can see that the form of the activity indulged in often contains a very accurate communication of the original breakdown or problem. They are by their very nature activities that precede symbolic functioning and therefore contain concrete forms of mental problems. This is the reason why narcissistic patients have great difficulty in symbolizing. For example, a woman who had been sexually abused by her own father for several years whilst a pre-pubescent child, felt driven to setting fires in her 8-year-old daughter's bedroom. In this way she projected the inflamed part of herself into an object, attempting to gain control over her own disturbing experience by projecting it entirely into the other, in this case her daughter, someone who most closely resembled herself at the age when it happened.

Pathological narcissism as manifested in the perversions occurs where the need to have absolute control over the object has been so great that the equivalent fantasy of the thumb, the rubber fetish for instance, becomes idealized. The pervert has identified a part of the self, or invested an action or behaviour as the good object, i.e., the transvestite in fantasy becomes the mother and the bad parts are projected outside into the external objects. Getting into the object, dressing up as a woman or, as in the case of a trans-sexual, "becoming a woman" takes over all the primary object's qualities, enviously taking all the good so that the patient/infant becomes the source of gratification, and any other object being the source of it has to be robbed and devalued, as with the transvestite's wife, or the arsonist's 8-year-old daughter. The victim is subjugated and forced to carry the unwanted aspects of the self.

There is enormous hostility against any awareness that life and goodness lie outside the self. Destructiveness therefore dominates, particularly in those whose early experience has been traumatic and impoverished. If a narcissistic patient was to become aware of his envy toward the object it would be tantamount to acknowledging that it was the source of gratification and was not a part of himself. This would be unbearable and the acknowledgement of separateness and dependency has to be defended against at all costs. In extreme pathological narcissism, as in the perversions, this knowledge has to be entirely avoided. This can mean absolute destruction of the other as an entity except as an object to have control over. Cruelty and hate have to dominate, e.g. a man who indulged in cottaging and cruising (that is, promiscuous homosexual sex in lavatories and public places) after five years of analysis came to feel that something he was getting from me was useful. There had been considerable diminishment of his perversion to the point where he no longer felt the need to find violent "rough trade" strangers with whom to be intimate. He was able to work without getting into fights and was developing a number of long-term friends whom he valued. Consequently his wish to deal with his destructive feelings through masochism intensified in the transference. After a weekend he came back to his Monday session and discovered to his "surprise" that the chairs usually in the waiting area were not there. He took this to mean that I did not care about him any more, so although it was raining heavily outside he decided to sit on the doorstep. I was surprised to discover that he was not in my new waiting room some few feet away from where the old waiting area had been. It was not until some time after I had found him on the step that he disclosed to me his reason for sitting outside.

We discovered that he had forgotten that I had told him I was making a change to my waiting area; he acknowledge that he had known and we were able to explore his reasons for forgetting. He angrily acknowledged his wish to set me up as a cruel uncaring analyst. His growing awareness of his need for me had led him to set things up so that I could be seen as entirely uncaring, his trust in me could then be proved to be unfounded and he could return to the inhuman environments he had previously frequented. At least he did not have expectations of any humanity there and would not be conned by unscrupulous analysts. This need to maintain a cruel and narrow-minded environment has been described by Brenman (1958) and Sohn (1985).

In severe forms of perversion such as paedophilia or sexual murder the need to destroy completely any goodness in the other is all- powerful. For instance a paedophile remembered his own abuse: whilst at a children's home. He ran away to London at the age of twelve and was picked up by a man who under the pretext of caring for him brutally buggered him and abandoned him. He could remember these awful experiences with all the attendant pain and anger, but was unable in any way to associate his own abuse with the violent sexual abuse he inflicted upon his twelve-year-old victims whom he would trap in a block of council flats. Thus he dealt with the memory of his own experience by negating the experience of the other. The other became merely a way of ridding himself of what was painful and bad for him, which could be sadistically and physically put in the victim. He would describe how aggrieved he was with his victims when enacting this abuse, whilst at the same time in another part of the session feeling tearful at the reminder of his own abandonment at the hands of his erstwhile saviours who had abused him.

As Bollas (Edward Glover Lecture, 1993) has pointed out, those who have had to annihilate large parts of themselves to survive can only feel alive when they are annihilating the other. The serial killer will describe in detail the sense of relief and pleasure at having total power over this victim because at the moment all the badness of the impoverishment is in the victim and not in himself. It is he who is in a position to annihilate other selves, and this gives him relief through the projection of his own psychic state into the other. It is this defence against the death instinct, which has primary envy at its source, that lies at the heart of all perverse activity.

This denial of the other as being the source of love and comfort leads the patient to act destructively. This destructiveness is a defence against the knowledge of the need for love. The more this knowledge has to be destroyed, the more the other has to be enslaved, marginalized and in the final scenario killed. The act of total destruction only occurs in extreme circumstances as the need for an object into whom to project the unwanted parts necessitates its survival. However, in the serial abuser or killer this has been circumvented.

In consideration of this, the patients' problems should be explored by means other than physical, lest we will be colluding with patients' delusional belief that changing reality will change them. The pressure to alter thinking and collude with these patients, who often threaten suicide, is great. Yet, as with other forms of disturbance, physical treatment, although at first appearing fashionable, may be disproved later on. However, the case of the current fashion for surgical treatment is irreversible.

Mr D—Skirting around the issue

In a first diagnostic interview with Mr D, there was an enormous pressure to collude with his view of reality. He was thin and effeminate looking, rather camp in manner, like a woman slightly older than his age. A sort of rag trade type. He was dressed as a man. In his letter to the Clinic he had signed himself ambiguously as Teri and had used a letter heading establishing that he was a director of an organization that enabled professionals to deal with violence in their work.

He came to the point in a straightforward way, saying that he had come to terms with being a woman and had booked his appointment with the surgeon but wanted somewhere he could think about the important step that he was taking. He felt that the Gender Dysphoria Clinic was hooked on the idea that it was a straightforward gender question whereas he was aware it could be that he was a woman in a man's body or it could be to do with a problem with masculine figures. He had read the books and knew of the theories and probably thought he knew already where I stood in relation to these matters. I said that it felt as if he were saying that he was aware of differing perspectives, he was even aware of what I already thought. I wondered if this certainty he appeared to have something to do with his problem of not knowing what my agenda might be in relation to him.

He had thought that I might be a woman. He put this down to the problem he has with masculine figures in general. He told me he was an only child and his mother was wonderful, totally accepting of him as he was, and had even entertained and enjoyed going out with his homosexual partners. In photos he was always next to his mother whereas male figures were always distant. I mentioned his father and how distant he seemed; he grimaced, saying his father had been a cruel despot who had beaten both him and his mother and had turned to alcohol. He was now totally cut off and estranged from his father and "good riddance to him". He gave an idyllic account of how nice life had been between his mother and himself since father had left.

He moved quickly to the present and his work. He said that he had his own counselling practice although he had not done a training as such, previous therapy had always encouraged him to come out as himself and he now combined what he had learnt there with gender questions about gay and lesbian issues. It created a picture of a trans-sexual presiding over a world of equal opportunity where all things were equal and with himself as the great egalitarian. Anyone who challenged this was a fascist. I was the unremitting analytic dictator. He had already let me know that he thought Freud was a bit backward in relation to gender. I had a bizarre vision of a man leading a group on violence, gradually turning into a woman. He did not consider that this would present many difficulties.

I said that he seemed to have moved quite easily from talking about his absent father to his position as a counsellor dealing with gender issues and violence, both issues that he had told me he might be interested in exploring with me. I wondered if this was a common experience, that of not having something and with little pain actually trying to become or own it, meaning that one way of dealing with his own confusion was to somehow become an expert in helping other people with theirs. He was coming to see me for possible help in thinking about these issues but was telling me how good he was at advising others.

He then in quite a different tone explained to me various ideas on gender identity. I was an idiot and he was the expert. He said that he was and had always been gay even though he had also had heterosexual experiences. However, he was very aware that he did not want to grow up to be an old man. I had obvious thoughts about his wish to dis-identify with his father, wanting to castrate himself as a way of getting rid of his old man. He felt he was getting old and would be 40 soon and it would be too late. I thought it was as if he was talking about the fact that he would be unable to have children but what he thought he would give birth to would be a new him or her. He agreed he knew he couldn't be a real woman but even if he was he wouldn't have children anyway.

Throughout this I was made out to be the tough psychoanalyst dressed up in my theories. It was I who was "skirting around the issue". I was told that a penis could be got rid of without much problem or remorse. There was a lot of confusion in the session surrounding his identity; it was consistently felt to shift and the goal-posts were moved on many occasions. He was himself a therapist counsellor who was advising others on gender problems and violence. The basic message seemed to be: if I castrate myself then it is all right, but if you do not accept this then you are attacking, violating and mutilating my reality. Thus he dealt with his own confusion by projecting it.

I said to him that he had come here at one level to be able to think about things but that this did not provide the certainty that he could get from other approaches to his problem. He described his experience of his previous therapist who had become pregnant after seeing him for one year. He thought he had been robbed and began a course of electrolysis. He saw this as the beginning of his move to become a woman leading on to contacting the Gender Dysphoria Trust. I said in a way he was letting me know that he had felt robbed and this had led him to run to other means of trying to help himself. He agreed and said he felt that the Gender Dysphoria Trust had accepted the whole fantasy about cutting off parts of the self. I said he had been talking about how robbed and confused he had felt and that he turned to electrolysis on his body to cope with these feelings. He was able in the interview to acknowledge that changing one's body was not necessarily a satisfactory way of changing one's mind or dealing with painful feelings.

The session was full of this type of thing. He told me that his fantasy of being with a man whilst masquerading as a woman was that the other person would not know. He had a male friend who was a "female" prostitute and his male clients did not know, thus he projected his confusion unknowingly, if that is possible, into the unconscious of the other person, reversing the confusing messages of his mother that he feels he has had to contain through identification.

The other man becomes an unconscious participant in a homosexual act. Thus he has all the knowledge and the infantile position of not having knowledge is taken up by the man who is relating to a woman who is in reality male. Hs own confusion as a child left in a world with his mother, with father absent is reversed. He becomes the mother, getting inside her body and taking over all the primary objects qualities, giving them to himself and then he is in a position to seduce men. By enacting the seductive relationship that he felt he had had with his mother, he has dealt with his loss of father by becoming a woman [his mother] by emasculating himself, but gaining a man [his father] as a lover. This situation with all its attendant fears has forced him to give up all masculine identity.

This last clinical description is an illustration of some of the ideas discussed by Hakeem (2006, this volume) in his discussion of transsexualism. As with his patients, for my patient, what appears to be a rigid idea of being a stranger in one's own body is in fact a desperate attempt to deal with emotional conflicts without having the mental capacity to do so. In such circumstances what is then turned to is the body, or perhaps more accurately, what one remains with is the body, one's own in this case, others' bodies in the case of other patients.

CHAPTER TWELVE

Ethical problems treating paedophile patients

John Woods

> You cannot do psychotherapy with someone who has a loaded gun.
>
> Attr. Donald Winnicott

This chapter engages with the debate over the difficult issue of confidentiality in the clinical relationship, and explores the ethical ramifications of undertaking psychotherapeutic work with a patient who may pose a risk to children. Contrasts between adult and child psychotherapy provide a context for this debate. A specific case is described where the patient's need to regress in a safe place (the therapeutic relationship) has to be set against the recognition of external reality. A framework is proposed whereby an agreement may be made about the limits to the confidentiality, so that the analytic work has a secure base. This link with external reality is seen in the light of Ogden's theory of the "analytic third" (Ogden, 1966), which symbolically provides a fathering function that can modify a potentially pathogenic mother/infant relationship.

Introduction: the question of confidentiality

In his long-running and consistent support for total confidentiality Christopher Bollas maintains that "... the analytic instrument could not exist without complete freedom of thought ..." When such freedom is curtailed, as Bollas perceives it is by recent US legislature that requires therapists to report suspicions of child sexual abuse, then the work of psychotherapy is made impossible. Despite an intention to protect children and vulnerable people, the laws that deny the right to confidential treatment have ultimately, according to Bollas, damaged the public good. Thus, he says, clinics for sexual deviants have disappeared and experienced psychotherapists have abandoned working with such patients (Bollas, 2003, p. 167). These points are made in a special issue of the *British Journal of Psychotherapy*, where Bollas and colleagues propose that psychoanalytic psychotherapy needs to strengthen its boundaries and deter any form of mandatory reporting. However, most current codes of ethics, for example that of the British Association of Psychotherapists, make provision for special circumstances in which serious harm can, and should be, prevented by breaking confidentiality. And as anyone working in the public sector will testify, expectations are certainly increasing that therapists should readily make available any information generated by a psychotherapeutic treatment.

It is difficult perhaps to have a coherent legislation that applies to all situations; there are many differences to be taken into account between public and private work, not least the question of who is paying for treatment. If a therapist is working within an organization that is providing treatment he or she must abide by that organization's code of ethics, which is most likely to be in compliance with the Children Act of 1989: this states that the duty of care to children overrides that of patients (Sher, 2003, p. 140). Thus there is an overarching debate that therapists cannot avoid. The question of whose interests are being served relates also to more profound issues, such as the purpose and meaning of psychotherapy. On the one hand an important principle of psychodynamic treatment is to enable the patient to speak of everything, including that which is forbidden elsewhere. The therapist cannot be a completely disinterested party since it is hardly possible to be neutral about child abuse. The purpose must be that the patient should receive the help which may be available nowhere else. The risk that such confidentiality might be perverted into collusion and secrecy and so prevent change, is offset by any given therapist's interpretive powers and faith in the therapeutic process. In the case of a sex offender the therapist is in effect hopeful of a "cure" to the patient's sexual deviancy. Lapses might be seen as expectable, or even necessary on the road to recovery. Reporting would in this view be destructive of the therapy, and if it happened would cause the *therapist* to be accused of being abusive, of identifying with an aggressor in society, harming a "vulnerable child" (in the form of the patient). A central tenet of forensic psychotherapy is the concept of the victim hidden within the perpetrator (Van Velsen, 1997, p. 160). It is not surprising therefore that this question of confidentiality has lately given rise to such intense debate in the profession, particularly as it applies to such an emotive subject as child abuse, and the possible involvement of therapists in unethical situations.

Fred and Mary West's son was convicted and sentenced to imprisonment for sex with a 14-year-old girl. This was a man who in his childhood witnessed his parents raping and killing family members as well as people they picked up from the street, and little attempt was made to understand the meaning of his own offence (Johann Hari's report, *The Independent*, 27th October 2004). A court of law can consider only the crime presented before it, in order to implement their task of protecting children from further abuse. But this case also highlights a need to look beyond the overt facts and to consider what produces an abuser. Research shows that a perpetrator is bound to have a history of abuse against him, though it may not be as dramatic as in that of the West family (Bentovim & Davenport, 1992; Bentovim, 1993). *Developments in Forensic Psychotherapy* (Cordess & Cox, 1996) shows how work with the suppressed victim in the offender helps release the vicious cycle of abuse. To reach that victim there will need to be an undoing of the defensive system of the abuser, which will necessitate a regression of some kind. It is particularly in this context, of the perpetrator's history of having been a victim, that reporting will be seen as an act of violence to the therapy, and a repetition of the abuse against the patient. It is crucial therefore to have some assessment of the regression, and whether it is likely to lead to change or not. This question is returned to later.

Confidentiality as a metaphor for protection against trauma

If, as Bollas (2003, p. 167) suggests, psychotherapy is "the most profoundly private relation yet established in western Culture", then much depends on what the therapist brings to this situation, at a personal as well as professional level. As a child psychotherapist I soon learned not to take anything for granted when embarking upon psychotherapy. A young person's environment has to be considered in all aspects, before attempting to create a therapeutic setting. One would not for example commence therapy for a child whose home environment was abusive or neglectful, or whose education had broken down, without making sure these things have received attention. Boundaries remain constant issues during the course of treatment. As well as how much confidentiality is appropriate, there is sometimes the question of whether or how much the therapist permits violent or dangerous behaviour. There is a duty of care to which the child therapist becomes accustomed where the patient must above all be kept safe, and this may be as much from himself, or herself, as from others. I have discussed elsewhere a systemic framework for psychodynamic work with young people who have committed sexual offences (Woods, 2003). Although here in the role of adult therapist I cannot ignore the perspective of the child's needs. Paula Heimann famously referred to her adult patients as "children-no-longer", something that could be said to apply particularly to those whose symptomatology is so bound up with children. The rules of the setting may change according to the patient's developmental stage, but there are some important connections that the "abuser" has to make with the abused child within himself.

The setting to serve the task

In a child's treatment there are obvious reasons for striving to maintain predictability. The disturbed child's inner world is disturbing as much to the child as his behaviour may be to adults. For that inner world to be communicated the immature person needs above all to feel secure in the knowledge that traumatic experiences of intrusion, abuse or abandonment will not be repeated. Thus a contained setting makes possible the exploration of such fears and pains in the transference and counter-transference. The term "therapeutic setting" implies also something inherently therapeutic about the setting (Hartnup, 1999). And "therapeutic" implies healing, though for long periods this may seem remote. Therapists may well be disappointed to the point of despair if they feel they are failing to provide a healing experience for patients or clients.

As someone who speaks from a great deal of experience of working with young people, Peter Wilson warns against unrealistic notions of cure. He speaks about the "primary task" of psychotherapy that helpfully defines "what" we are doing, rather than how we feel we should be doing.

> The primary task of the psychotherapist is to ensure conditions of work that facilitate communication, and enable both therapist and patient to observe and think about what is happening between them. The concept of a therapeutic setting refers to everything that forms the background in which psychotherapy takes place.
>
> [Wilson 1991, p. 260]

Perhaps this concept of background can be extended to the idea of an ethical framework. The basis of most ethical codes is that we should act in the patient's best interests. How can reporting on a patient's transgressions be in his interests? Some therapists maintain that the welfare of people other than their own patient, including children, is not their business. And yet the law says that if you know that your patient is abusing children, and do nothing, you are participating. Does this dilemma destroy the treatment? Is it possible, in Wilson's terms, to observe and think about what is happening between patient and therapist, against the background of tolerating child abuse?

Compromise, though a dirty word for some, is perhaps the only way to maturity, said Winnicott (1988, p. 137). With the treatment of adults there is more room for manoeuvre. A middle way of confidentiality is proposed by some writers on the subject. Rob Hale (2003, p. 139) clearly considered it an achievement of his working party that they established "a statutory duty to consider *whether* to disclose". A way through the maze is also proposed by Mannie Sher who discusses the current thinking on patient/professional partnership. He recommends a pragmatic approach. Given that there can be no absolute level of confidentiality, psychotherapists should be prepared to disclose when appropriate (2003, p. 142). In this way patients and therapists can be given the opportunity to decide together on the sharing of information, without either being bound by a fundamental rule. If no agreement can be reached then there can be no working together. Such an approach allows for differences between therapists, but is no easy solution, because more is going on than usually meets the eye.

Psychodynamics in the treatment alliance

Chris McKenna, writing on ethical pressures on the working alliance, shows that we ignore unconscious processes at our peril. The "acting out" of feelings may be undertaken in hidden ways, despite (or perhaps because of) their passionate intensity. McKenna alerts us to the unconscious "identifications" that may develop in spite of the conscious, working alliance. But the situation is complicated because it is from that "dark, experiential place", as McKenna puts it, that interpretation flows. This is to say that the unspoken dynamics between therapist and client become the material that has to be understood. When they are enacted in a non-thought-out way, as in the example given by McKenna of a patient of Masud Khan's, the results are disastrous. Wynne Godfrey, one of Khan's ex-patients, publicized many instances of breaches of boundaries all of which point to the needs of the therapist outweighing those of the patient. McKenna quotes Godfrey as saying that he felt he was attempting to save the therapist (McKenna, 2003, p. 52). This is reminiscent of the incest victim who is burdened with the unsatisfied needs of the incestuous parent. McCarthy (1988) identified this as one of the main dynamics of incest, one that leaves the incest victim with such feelings of hate. Therapists working with patients of any age must first and foremost examine the reasons for our actions, including interpretation, and ask in whose interests is this? Our behaviour will inevitably be in our own interests to some extent, but we need to be clear in what way this is so. We do have to earn a living, we are interested in complex tasks, we do have a need, more or less conscious and no doubt from our own early experience, to repair our own inner world. But if we have to be always helpful, when we begin to entertain notions of cure, rescue, saving people, then alarm bells start to ring.

McKenna (2003) has given a useful discussion of the predicament of seeking too much to help. He shows how notions of healing may be full of pitfalls. Not all can be predicted because at the outset neither patient nor therapist knows quite what they are letting themselves in for. He shows how codes of ethics, whilst necessary in order to provide limits as to what can be expected from the therapist, actually do little to resolve real ethical dilemmas, such as the difficulty of paternalism, "the therapist knows best". This error can lead to interpretations that the patient cannot accept. Awareness of this problem is highlighted in the work of Anne Alvarez (1997), who has explored in great detail the timing of interpretations and the need for the therapist to find ways of responding to that which may be still traumatic for the patient. Failure to find tolerable means of communication leaves both feeling misunderstood, helpless and alone. A therapist could stay completely within codes of ethics, and yet do nothing of value for their patient. McKenna warns against "absolutism", which, like fundamentalism in religion inhibits thought, takes us away from the uniqueness of an individual, and against the autonomy for which they may be striving in their therapy. The values that therapists hold in practice are therefore at least as important as the codes, which tend to be "thou shalt not". Agreements about a contract for therapy, unlike codes, are a reflection of what kind of working relationship may be possible. So if it is recognized that confidentiality is not just a matter of rules, then the specific needs of patients can be taken into account.

Provision for therapeutic regression

Donald Winnicott (1954) pointed out the tendency in psychoanalytic psychotherapy for the setting to evoke regression. Whereas the reliability of the time, place, physical conditions, attention of the therapist etc might symbolize for the neurotic patient something like maternal love, for some other patients (whether they be called psychotic, borderline, personality disordered, or just plain deprived), the treatment setting becomes indistinguishable from the desired state itself. This results in excessive demands for contact with the therapist, or its opposite, a phobic avoidance of the setting in its function of regulating emotional contact. For Winnicott the appropriate expression of the therapist's hate was in the ending of sessions, the requirement of the fee, etc; these counterbalance unrealistic demands that the therapist compensate for failed parenting. In tolerating his own hate the therapist reproduces, but then transforms, the original parents' failure, which was a hate that could not be borne.

Michael Balint identified different kinds of regression; he distinguished that which is necessary for the building of new and more effective adaptations to reality, from a malignant regression, which was akin to an addictive relationship with an ultimately frustrating object. Throughout his writing he disputed the notion of an intrapsychic or "individual" psychology, being much more in favour of a "two-person" view of the interaction of psychotherapy. For example, in an illustration of benign regression, Balint (1968, p. 143) shows how a patient's silence was treated not as a resistance or an avoidance of contact but in that particular case as a manifestation of an inner process of emotional change; the analyst had to leave the patient alone, as he put it, "to get on with his inner world". This was a person who as a child always had people telling him what to do. Balint reports a moment when a new experience was provided, not by the analyst's intention to heal, or to cure, so much as by clarity in the task of exploring the meaning of what was occurring in the session. Had the analyst tried to be "helpful" and told the patient what to do, or how to be, then a possible "new beginning" for the patient's emotional integration would have been lost. In this sense the analyst provides something more akin to an environment in which the patients may learn about themselves. Balint speaks metaphorically about a perception of the therapist at the level of part object, that is when the patient is regressed to a point in development at which the other is not perceived as a whole person, but something like a substance, such as water that is needed for someone to be able to swim, or the earth, needed for someone to walk. Transference interpretations in this situation, for example, that the patient may be feeling that the therapist is like an oppressive father, or abandoning mother, may seem irrelevant to the patient, and therefore of little value. At certain stages it is more important that the therapist function as an externally real object, rather than as a vehicle for the exploration of fantasy. This would be consistent with recognition of the reality both of child abuse and of the law that exists to prevent it.

Clinical illustration

Session 1

Mr J, in his fifties, has been in three-times-a-week psychotherapy for two years. This is an interchange that took place at some point in the first few months. He arrived as usual on time for the first session after the weekend. He entered and lay on the couch. After a short pause he said,

"I don't know whether to say this. I don't know if you are going to disapprove."

I said nothing.

After a pause he went on to say he had seen such a happy child walking with his mum in the street on the way here. He was holding her hand and chatting away. The child had a beautiful smile and seemed so carefree.

"Just as you would have wished to be," I said.

"Some hope," he said, bitterly, "I can't even bring myself to tell you for fear you will take it the wrong way. The more I say I won't do anything, the more you might think I'm covering up. I don't have any thoughts about that child—I mean anything you would be worried about. But I can't help the feelings." (*Silence.*) "And you can't help them either." (*Slight flash of anger here, quickly corrected.*) "I'm inflicting this on you, this insoluble problem. There is nothing to be done, I'm a hopeless case. Why don't you give up on me? Give your time to someone more deserving." (*Silence.*)

I say, "So it seems I could never be that mother who makes the child so carefree?"

"My mother? What a disaster."

There was a short pause and I realized he was weeping quietly.

"You know I really did love her. It was just that she . . . there was such a barrier . . ."

(*Silence.*)

> I say, "And now it seems the barrier is between you and me where you feel I should not bother with you . . ."
>
> (*Silence.*)
>
> "I dreamt, oh, I don't know if I can bear to tell you this. It is so appalling." (*He squirmed on the couch.*) "I dreamt I was in a bath full of shit. I can hardly bear to think of it, it is so appalling. And you must be disgusted even to hear of it!"
>
> I said, "I could be disgusted, unless I felt that you are also telling me how much you need to be cleaned up."
>
> "But aren't you disgusted by me? I am always surprised you should even bother seeing me."
>
> After a pause he went on: "But you're right. I need cleaning up. The trouble is it's always so . . .".
>
> And he went on to tell for the first time about his soiling himself as a child at boarding school, where he was not only excruciatingly ashamed but had to endure the somewhat less than sympathetic cleaning up by care staff, as well as contempt from other children

Mr J had sought help ostensibly for problems of depression and suicidal thoughts following the death of a close friend, a younger man, T, who was an artist and drug addict. But it soon emerged that he had serious obsessive/compulsive symptoms, of excessive cleanliness, rituals and checking. These seemed related to his paedophilia which was suppressed, and had not been acted upon for some years. He declined the psychiatrist's suggestion of medication, but took up an alternative offer of being referred for psychotherapy. An only child, his family background was dominated by a depressed mother who eventually committed suicide when Mr J was 19. From an over-close relationship, remembering her being in bed all the time, often with him, he was abruptly separated from her when he was sent to boarding school aged eight, where he was terrified and lonely. His father was described as remote, "a complete stranger". There was no history of overt sexual abuse against Mr J, though the physicality of his mother was described as overwhelming, being repelled by seeing her naked, by her body smells and so forth. Shortly after going to boarding school he was told that his parents were splitting up, which he recalled as "devastating". He had always thought he was indifferent to his mother's death, did not go to the funeral, and never cried. He drifted in adolescence, with little education and no satisfaction in his career. However he worked hard, taking refuge in tasks he always felt to be menial, and made a success of himself in a cleaning business. In his 20s he was targeting and paying children, waifs and strays in central London, for mutual masturbation. He was caught on one such occasion, and received a warning by the police. From that time on he lived a completely "celibate" existence refraining from sexual activity of any kind, apart from rare and joyless masturbation. For twenty years he had been dependent on T who was idealized, and had an apparently happy marriage, despite being a drug addict. There were erotic feelings, unexpressed, in the attachment to T who seemed to know about and to tolerate Mr J's paedophilia in an unspoken way; in so doing T may have helped prevent acting out. The bereavement was complex, since part of Mr J's acute depression was anxiety that no-one else would bear him, coupled with what we found out shortly after treatment began, a fear that without his friend his paedophilic behaviour may recur.

This case presents ethical dilemmas, some of which are rooted in counter-transference. Like most therapists who have worked with those who have been abused, I know that many abusers walk free. Victims of their crimes lose faith not only in the law, but in there being any justice in the adult world. I could certainly be disgusted by what Mr J has done. When I first met him I was reasonably convinced by his appeal for help, but in taking on the responsibility of treating him, would it be with an unconscious intention of making him suffer? Or was I compensating for this in myself by making excuses, as if to say "poor man; there but for the grace of God, go I!" And more worryingly, if he were to change and be released from persecuting guilt, would he no longer be abstinent? These questions come to a head over the specific and practical ethical problem of confidentiality in the setting. It was clear to me I could work only with ongoing consultation. When setting up treatment he agreed to my consulting with others, and to my using his material in order to further the understanding of people with his problem, whilst preserving his anonymity. He further agreed that if he were to interfere with a child he would report himself, or I would. This of course does not sit easily within usual practice which prohibits the therapist from taking anything outside the setting, but the BAP's code of ethics, as referred to above, as well as those of most other organizations, make it clear that the safety of children would override the rule of confidentiality. This understanding between us at the outset enabled me to feel that I need neither condone nor condemn. In a public service establishment such as the Portman Clinic this kind of support network is normally in place. In private practice where in-depth treatment (i.e., more frequent sessions) is more likely to be available, the equivalent has to be made possible. With this structure it is possible to put aside a need to "cure" the patient, which could easily be a compensation for another desire, to punish.

Mr J quickly became emotionally dependent on the therapy and seemed to collapse for a few months, being unable to work. The regression was manageable, and fairly well contained in the therapy. Part of it was the still strong grief reaction to the loss of his close friend, the drug addict. But the pain was also derived from earlier abandonings, going to boarding school, which had then been closely followed by his "world falling apart" as he put it when his parents split up. He became aware during treatment of long denied feelings about his mother's suicide. We were able to link these experiences with his adolescent sexual development in which the erotic fixation on pre-pubescent boys seemed partly to be a wish to regain the childhood he felt had been taken from him. It also represented a refusal to grow and separate from a mother towards whom consciously he felt bitterness and rage. Mr J had internalized a parental couple where there was little life-giving interaction. His attachment to the treatment came to represent both a refuge from the world of terrifying loss and also a place where his self-loathing and emotional pain could be located and made tolerable.

Session 2

After a year or so in treatment he began to work part time and became more sociable in his everyday life. In this session he had been telling me of a pleasant evening he had spent with friends.

"Seeing them all made me realize how different I am; they have relationships, I mean they hold hands with someone, they live with someone. People care about them. God, I sound so pathetic."

I said, "You expect me also to dismiss your longing for contact."

"No, I don't want you to think I don't appreciate what you are doing for me . . . I mean I do, it's just that . . . well, you do seem to perhaps care when I'm here, but then when it's time to go, you say 'Right, time's up, off you go,' and then it's 'next please', and forget about me! God, I hate myself, for sounding so . . . spoilt." (*Pause.*) "I think you have saved my life, and I sound so ungrateful, perhaps my life wasn't particularly worth saving . . . It's just that I crave some physical contact, and I can only imagine it with a boy. You know I won't do anything. I know, I really know it would be destructive. It would be no good, I don't want to fuck a boy, or have him fuck me, I want to be held, and hold someone. It just can't work with an adult, I don't know what to do sexually with an adult."

I said, "So you are trying to distinguish physical affection with a particular sort of sex, called fucking, in an abusive way."

"I actually don't know what it would be like, really. I don't know what it is like, to be held, to be kissed. You must be so bored by me, whinging on like this! I sound like a two-and-a-half-year old!"

I said, "I guess that must have been when you were last kissed by your mother."

"I couldn't stand her kissing me, her smell, and . . . but . . . I couldn't stand to be without her . . ." (*Silence.*) "I can just feel . . ." (*Pause.*) "I think I just felt her kiss on my cheek. You probably think I'm making it up."

I said, "So it feels like I would attack the moment when the child in you was kissed by mother. Like a father who would not allow it?"

"He was never there."

I said, "He was never there physically, just as I cannot be there to physically make up for the lack of love."

He wept quietly.

I said nothing but was conscious of the tragedy of his development that had meant he was cut off from physical love and contact perhaps forever. I felt there was little I could do and felt tearful at the inevitability of this moment of awareness.

Discussion

Mr J's early relationships and subsequent difficulties can be understood in the light of Mervyn Glasser's theory of the "core complex"; this shows how the symptomatology of sexual perversion develops from a need to control the object in order to prevent traumatic states of being either overwhelmed or isolated (Glasser, 1964). This in turn originates, according to Glasser, from a primary maternal relationship that has been experienced as over-close and abandoning by turns. At times I have wondered if Mr J's mother looked upon her baby as providing some consolation in an unhappy marriage, and so

Mr J would have conceived of himself as an attempted cure to his mother's despair. I have also speculated that she may herself have been affected by experiences of child sexual abuse, but there is no historical information as to this. It was as if her child was the embodiment of unintegrated sexuality. At any rate the attachment to mother was eroticized albeit for him in a repellent way, and independence felt impossible, just as he could not separate himself from his own infantile sexuality.

The absence of an effective father in the family life of the future sexual pervert is just as significant as the quality of the maternal relationship, points out Glasser; it is the father who would normally facilitate an appropriate masculine development (Glasser, 1988). The role of father is central to the understanding of sexual perversion as one that can modify the mother/infant dysfunction (or should have done). It is often thought that fathering complements mothering by standing for limits (Trowell & Etchegoyen, 2002, p. 23). The father's "No" is a much-needed protection against omnipotence, and the consequent terrors in child development (Johns, 2002, p. 188). In representing the external world, whilst recognizing the impulses and desires of the child, the father thereby modifies the child's internal world. Mr J's treatment therefore depended upon a symbolic fathering where external reality was given as much weight as the more nurturing provision of a safe space for the exploration of his internal reality.

By the second session described above I found that I was more able to think in a reflective fashion, and this was rather similar to that which Ogden (1966), borrowing a term from Bion, describes as *reverie*. Initially I had been a sort of policeman/father who controls and stops the patient from abusing children. As we worked on the representation in paedophilia of the disordered mother/infant bond, I became a different sort of father, one who comes between him and mother in a more life-giving way. Ogden talks of the *analytic third*, as the product of what happens between therapist and patient. The setting of this particular therapy was constructed to include child protection, an external consideration. Some analytic therapists would not include this, and would offer total confidentiality. Others like myself would feel too limited by that, and need a kind of boundary that gives the freedom to relate to the outside world. Such a permeable boundary may lead, as in this case, to an analytic third, over and above the therapeutic dyad. What might have been seen as an external demand was then experienced as a necessary contribution from father, to separate the child from infantile omnipotence by introducing social reality. Paradoxically this has been the key, I believe, to open the door of his inner world. In addition to the I and Thou of therapist and patient, therefore, there is this third element; sometimes it is the world *out there*, the patient's existence in the world with all its dangers for him, and there is also the third *in here*, the one which is created, as Ogden shows, between therapist and patient. Thus the external did not inhibit the analytic work; the meaning of the dream for example was changed in the telling, it seemed, from one of horror (especially to someone so obsessed with cleanliness) to one of truth, because in relation to his therapist he could experience his need to be cleansed. Similarly in the later session there was interplay between us when he spoke of his craving for physical affection. There was still the anger, humiliation and shame but this was gradually changing into an acceptance of loss, and the reality of that with the memory of his mother's kiss.

The profound sense of loss conveyed by this patient affected me more deeply than similar feelings conveyed by those patients who have been abused rather than become an abuser. Winnicott (1947, p. 195) says that the therapist can only help a patient with things they have reached in themselves. Whilst it is not difficult to identify with loss, nor the experience of forbidden sexual relations, to renounce one's whole sexual life is something more painful to imagine. I was left with respect for him, rather than the contempt I might have had. Although he may never be "cured" there is nevertheless much that is achievable in terms of his other symptoms. Work can continue as the professional role contains the therapist's own revulsion and impulse to condemn. Struggling not to obey the desires to abuse, this patient had been seriously depressed, enslaved to his obsessional symptoms, persecuted by thoughts that the world would hate him, and contemplating suicide. He had always known that to sexually seduce a child would be a destructive act unacceptable to himself, but the fear and guilt that was stopping him also took away any sense of his life being worth anything. For years he had managed to deny the truth of himself, always in fear that if the other knew him he would be rejected. It has emerged during the treatment that T, his "dearest friend", was perhaps not so selflessly devoted to Mr J as imagined, but was instead a steady drain on Mr J's financial and emotional resources. The attachment to an exploitative drug addict has now been seen, more sadly, deriving from the primary relationship with a self-destructive and therefore depriving mother. Hence also the conviction in his transference that I am unable to bear him and would rather give my time elsewhere.

To pursue technical questions in relation to counter-transference a little further, the question arises whether it might have been therapeutic for me to respond to his need for physical contact, by touching, or holding him? Some therapeutic approaches might allow for this. But where would the boundary have been drawn? Should I have stopped there, or provided the kiss he so yearned for? Who would this have been for?—For the patient, who might have an experience of someone who could bear him and even offer a physical comfort for his pain?—Or for the therapist to feel that nobly he had overcome his own resistance to the revulsion he had felt against this man? Supposing it were done, would the patient have moved from his massive internal prohibition against physical/erotic contact? Would he then be coming to therapy for physical consolation rather than grappling with his difficulty in having an adult physical relationship? There is no means of knowing if physically holding him for example would produce the internal change he needs. But if he is given the space to express what is happening in his internal world (just as Balint's restraint gave the patient an opportunity to experience himself in a new way), Mr J is reorienting himself to his own life and finding what is possible as well as impossible in relation to others. This needs to be done in his own mental—and therefore physical—space. And there is much work to be done, on the fantasy life that underlies the paedophilia.

Finally, is it ethical to use this man's treatment as a kind of research project to learn about the psychodynamics of paedophilia, to discuss technical questions and publish findings as I have done here? Despite his permission, am I perhaps expressing, as Winnicott (1947) might have said, my *hate* of him, my need to reject and separate myself from his tortured world, and a bit of self-aggrandisement to boot? Again, it is the protection of the setting that enables not only the task to be preserved, but also the therapist to avoid either condoning or condemning. The setting provides a certain neutrality, which is different from indifference. The *ethical* setting enables the treatment to take place by freeing the therapist to function. It is obviously in the patient's best interests that he be helped stay away from children, but the work should be able to go deeper, and its significance requires debate with colleagues. The safety net of reporting is there so that the therapist will not be left alone with the knowledge that children are being abused. Such an external reference point also perhaps has a reparative significance in relation to the early maternal relationship. Though it is not known if his mother had been sexually abused and gone on to use her child as a sexual object, it is clear that she must have been so alone with her unhappiness that she killed herself. In Mr J's therapy he has the experience of being with someone who is *not* left alone with intolerable feelings: symbolically he finds a mother, it could be said, who has also the presence of a father who can protect, and make possible a relationship with the outside world.

Conclusion

Hester McFarland Solomon has put forward the notion of an ethical attitude which is far more than just the avoidance of rule-breaking. Coming from a Jungian perspective she talks about self-realization and the integration of the shadow side of the personality. Emotion and thought, she says, struggle together to reach a state of *ethical discernment* (Solomon, 2002, p. 25). She draws from neuroscience to show how mutuality and atunement between mother and infant are crucial to the development of the infant's sense of self. Ultimately, she says the ethical capacity will derive from these early, albeit instinct-driven exchanges. An ethical attitude develops into "an ability to transcend narcissistic considerations and to truly apprehend the other". This could be proposed both as an ultimate aim, and an immediate goal of psychotherapy—to recognize and relate to the truth of the other. There is no need therefore for the paedophile patient to be "cured" of his sexual orientation to children; rather he can be helped to develop an understanding of himself *in relation to his social world*, with all that entails, i.e., the impossibility of enacting his sexual desires. This increased emotional connectedness to himself will allow him to be aware of something in the other as much as in himself, i.e. a child who should not be abused.

CHAPTER THIRTEEN

The forensic network and the internal world of the offender[1]

Thoughts from consultancy work in the forensic sector

Richard Davies

> . . . the Child is looking for something, somewhere and failing to find it seeks elsewhere, when hopeful.
>
> [Winnicott 1956, p.306]

> . . . when the environment does not understand the inner significance of antisocial behaviour, such behaviour is likely to become aggravated.
>
> [Limentani 1966, p.277]

Introduction

The view is taken in this paper that professionals who deal with offenders are not free agents but potential actors who have been assigned roles in the individual offenders' own re-enactment of their internal world drama. The professionals have the choice not to perform but they can only make this choice when they have a good idea of what the role is they are trying to avoid. Until they can work this out they are likely to be drawn into the play, unwittingly and therefore not unwillingly. Because of the latter, if the pressure to play is not anticipated then the professional will believe he is in a role of his choosing. Unfortunately, initially, only a preview of the plot is available in the somewhat cryptic form of the offence. If this is misunderstood then further opportunities to "preview" may arise through further offences but the behaviour may become worse. As long as the offending continues there is some hope, albeit diminishing, for the professional and thus for the offender whose internal drama is the subject for modification.

If some initial sense is made of the "assigned" role then time may be given to understand more, and further clues may be provided for encouragement. At the same time pressure will continue to be applied to play the assigned role. That is to say, accompanying the hope conveyed through the offence will also be an attack on hope.

It is also important to comment that it is not only the offender's internal drama that professionals are called upon to enact but also those more explicit scripts of their own organizations and central government. They will also be under pressure from themselves to re-enact their own dramas. Thus for example a professional who was adopted may experience great difficulties in working with a client who has just lost a parent. The professionals I refer to throughout have "clients", "patients", "suspects", "defendants" and "prisoners". For convenience I have settled on "client" and also for convenience, the masculine pronoun "he".

Case example

The following is an instance of how various professionals responded to a dangerous man who had been released from prison. It is an extreme case in terms of level of disturbance, chosen for what I believe to be its clear illustrative value. It is not, however, atypical, in my view, of how professionals can often respond. It is an actual case disguised sufficiently to protect confidentiality without detracting from the significant points. I have tried to outline the case as simply as possible.

This is a case in which I was asked to offer consultation to a probation officer. I was also provided retrospectively with some detailed information by others who had been involved.

Brief case details

A 43-year-old man was released from prison following a long sentence for committing two particularly vicious rapes of middle-aged women. He was only at liberty for twenty hours before he raped again. This time it was a pregnant woman who subsequently lost her child. He then went on to commit a violent sexual assault on an eleven-year-old girl. He was arrested with little difficulty shortly after and went on to serve another long sentence.

All the women lived alone. He had observed that the girl had been alone in a park for some hours before he attacked her. On the first occasion he was released without anywhere to live and had gone to his elderly mother who had refused to let him live with her. He had been considered too dangerous to release any earlier than was absolutely necessary; he was therefore deprived of the statutory parole supervision he would have received if released earlier. Following the second sentence he was again released at the latest possible date and therefore again without statutory supervision.[2] It had been recognized by all those who knew the case that it was not realistic to expect such a man to "survive" for very long outside prison and that the likelihood was that he would have to commit further offences; thus it had been implicitly accepted that: (a) people would have to be harmed, and (b) there was nothing anyone could do about it.

However, a female probation officer, with whom he had been in contact while in prison, took a serious interest in him and recognizing his dangerousness, organized a placement in a hostel, which catered for ex-prisoners. She agreed to provide liaison support. She did this against considerable resistance from her authority which was concerned to prioritize the numerous cases for which they were obliged to provide statutory supervision; there were few resources for "voluntary" supervision. The probation officer held her ground pointing out that an attempt to do something was seen as preferable to standing by and waiting for more rapes and assaults on women and children.

There was an element of hope in that the man was worried himself about further violence and had, in fact, asked if he could stay in prison. It was useful therefore that he was willing to co-operate voluntarily with the arrangements made by the probation officer, perhaps hoping that the hostel would have a prison-like regime.

The summary details of his history were that his father abandoned the family soon after the third child, a sister, was born; he was the second child. He reported no memory of his father. His mother remarried and two more girls arrived. This marriage also collapsed and mother raised the five children on her own. He described his mother as having been harsh and violent towards him and he had been frightened of her. He described having been singled out by her for harsh treatment while his elder brother, the first child, was treated well. He reported that since adolescence his sexual experiences had been largely homosexual. He was afraid of making normal advances to women because he thought they would reject and ridicule him.

The hostel, which had been arranged by the probation officer, accepted him in the knowledge that he was dangerous, particularly to women, and so arranged that he would be carefully monitored by the manager and deputy, both males. Female staff were to have minimal contact with him. It was known that he had withdrawn from group treatment in prison as he could not tolerate it and this was taken as an indication that he would require careful supportive management but without intensive counselling. The wish and the anxiety to know what he was thinking and feeling and where he was going, had to be resisted on the basis that it might provoke him to leave, or worse, provoke him into action. It would be difficult to resist the wish to know because the anxiety about him would be very high, both in relation to staff safety and that of the community.

The need for a constant awareness of his violence and to "hold on to the anxiety" and contain this on his behalf without expecting any fundamental change was central to the plan.

Within a week of the man's arrival the hostel manager had to go on extended sick leave and the deputy took over his role and became quickly entrenched in administration, thus considerably diminishing his monitoring role in relation to this man. The remaining staff members, who were all female, perhaps feeling that they had no option, agreed that one of them would offer him counselling on the basis that this might provide him with a positive experience of a woman. Somehow the original plan had already been subverted. The "unwitting actors" were already beginning to take on their "assigned" roles.

The probation officer was not told of the above sequence of events. Soon after, the man was seen by a hostel staff member standing outside a school near the hostel at the time children were due to leave. The male deputy dealt with it appropriately by telling the man he had been seen and warned him against going near the school. However, the deputy then withdrew into his administrative work and became inaccessible. It was later learned that the man continued to hang around schools and had been seen speaking to children.

As time went on his contact with the female worker increased, mainly at her instigation. Because of the collapse of the support framework this worker could not safely acknowledge her anxiety and later reported that she had found herself saying to the man that he was good looking and sexy and that he could easily find a girlfriend. She had been unwittingly drawn into a sado-masochistic situation. The man asked her if she would like to be his girlfriend. Without the proper support that would have both helped her to withdraw while simultaneously providing containment for the man, the worker compensated for that lack and fell into the role of both victim and tormentor. She was the "victim" by putting herself in that situation and the "tormentor" by appearing from this man's point of view to offer something and then to withdraw it. She began to see progress that didn't exist in the man. She talked with him alone at night in the hostel for long periods, often with no other staff members in the vicinity. She claimed that she did not feel afraid and felt sure that he would not be violent towards her. She later admitted that she had forgotten he had committed rape and remembered his offence as "an assault" of some kind. Something serious had clearly happened to her capacity to think and to remember, and also to the minds of the rest of the hostel staff and its management who had failed to notice what was happening.

Further events which occurred are stated in brief for clarity. The probation officer saw the problem and attempted to help the staff look at the dangerous position in which they had placed themselves and also the community they were seeking to protect. The female worker withdrew and the male deputy came back into the picture. At the same time, however, the probation officer had also been offering the man appointments at her office at night and then after she had seen him would walk alone to a dark car park. The man expressed fears of his compulsion to rape. The fact that he could say this was a measure of the degree to which he felt held in the minds of others. He perhaps experienced being taken more seriously than ever before in his life.

Paradoxically it became even more difficult to "hold him in mind" as the ability to think was in danger of being overwhelmed by the high level of anxiety that had been engendered. Extra male staff were urgently requested and the management committee provided agency staff, for twenty-four hours. Subsequently, the client received a letter from the management committee warning him that he was disrupting the hostel and costing them money and if he did not "behave" he would have to leave.

The client then began to express suicidal feelings that seemed easier for the staff to address than his rape warning. He was referred to a telephone counselling service that suggested he find a prostitute as an outlet for his aggression.

Around this time it was discovered that a female prison visitor who had seen him frequently during his sentence had renewed contact with him without the knowledge of her organization. She invited him to her house where he hit her several times and he then begged her to call the police. She refused and tried to persuade him to talk. He complained of feeling suicidal and ran to the local Samaritans who talked with him for several hours. Although he told them what he had done they could not help him to go to the police because no crime had been reported. He left and immediately took an overdose. He was admitted to hospital where they recorded that he was extremely depressed and at risk of suicide. They discharged him the next day. He returned to the hostel where he appeared very angry and frustrated. The probation officer referred him to a medium secure unit for assessment.

In spite of threats and protests the client attended for assessment at the secure unit. He explained that he had been out armed with a knife on the previous evening, had visited a prostitute and, unable to get an erection, had taken an overdose. He was admitted as a voluntary patient, discharging himself shortly after. Later he was detained under the Mental Health Act and, having been put on the "observation" ward, absconded. He rang a radio station confessing to rapes that he couldn't possibly have committed. The police tracked him down and arrested him but released him soon after as a "crank." Eventually, after further absconsions and complications about his status under the Mental Health Act, he was transferred to a special hospital.

Some observations

1. If the probation officer had not struggled against her own organization at the outset there would have been no plan of containment and it can be assumed that violent sexual offences would have quickly occurred if the man had simply been released into the community without any support.
2. The "available" men, like the man's father, disappeared very quickly, not to be replaced.

3. None of the women protected themselves properly and each, including the volunteer, attempted to draw him into the kind of close working relationship which had been contraindicated. They repeated for the man his experience of a sadistic mother with whom he had felt trapped. Subsequent to the breakdown of his homosexual defence in adolescence the only psychological route of escape open to him was sexualized violence.
4. Until the final event, all the institutions that exist to take disturbed people seriously (police, hospitals, prisons, secure units) let him go.
5. With the important exception of point 1, where the probation officer struggled usefully with her own organization and also with the hostel, a thinking "couple" was barely evident. Potential "couples" would have been: the hostel and its management committee; the other workers and their female colleague; the volunteer and her "parent" organization; the police and the Health Service; the probation officer and her supervisor.

Discussion

Why was there such a discrepancy between what was agreed and the way people acted?

If we maintain too close a focus on the professionals we risk seeing only what they "did" and commenting on what they could or should have "done" and we either conclude that they did their best or criticize them or their management. We may then, amongst other proposals, suggest regular supervision, with which few people would disagree. Equally, we may criticize the volunteer or her supervisor, and forget that a volunteer is somebody we ask to befriend someone; can we now ask her to un-befriend? We could criticize government for poor resources such that in residential provision, in particular, the most inexperienced, unqualified and unsupported staff predominate amongst those who look after the most seriously disturbed people in our society.

If something serious had occurred, as was highly possible, there would inevitably have been an inquiry that would have produced yet more guidelines about communication, vigilance and alarm systems. It would certainly have looked for people to hold accountable.

It would not however have touched upon the unconscious attack on the professionals' capacity to think—the essential prerequisite for liaison and vigilance. It would not have looked to understand how, with their thinking impaired, the professionals were vulnerable to the roles assigned to them from the man's internal world drama, through the processes of projection and projective identification.

When unsupported professionals become aware of behaving towards a client in a way they either dislike or feel they would like to disown, they too look for someone to blame. "Management" is a frequent target but equally so is the client.

A familiar phrase "He is manipulative" is often used (see Cox 1994 on manipulation). It is frequently used in a way which appears to attribute blame to the offender for making the professional feel manipulated such that "he stops me from thinking straight and gets me to do things for him"; "He gets people to collude with him and they get sucked in . . . he is very powerful". The offender stands accused of a further "offence".

Another sort of blaming occurs where the concept of "splitting" is sometimes (mis)used to describe something that the client *does* to two or more professionals to set them against each other to stop them working together. The client also is held responsible for "projecting his feelings into" people and making them feel "angry" or "untrusting".

If the client really is this powerful, however, we have to ask why does he bother to adopt the high-risk strategy of offending to achieve his objective?

If we turn to the professionals we hear of how they cannot think, or of how they feel impelled to do, say or feel things they later wished they hadn't. They may squabble amongst themselves and feel highly critical of each other and may refuse to speak to one another. In other words, professionals can often appear to be quite helpless and powerless and may retrospectively describe themselves in these terms. When they "discover" what has happened to make them feel uncomfortable they may blame the client and sometimes may even complain to him for what he has "done" to them. The action of the hostel management committee in writing to admonish the man was an example of this.

Yet while we know that this phenomenon occurs, how do we

come to think of somebody such as this man as being so psychologically powerful when we know how frightened he was of his violence and how his principal means of relating to the world was through futile acts of violence to women and children and through brief homosexual encounters with men? He would probably agree that it was because he felt so powerless on release from prison that he accepted the help offered.

Initially the professionals in this case would certainly have seen themselves as behaving as though they were in charge. Yet to an observer, the professionals in the hostel and elsewhere might be seen to be acting "as if" they were powerless and "as if" the client was directing the drama. However, the staff in the hostel were only able to begin to observe this phenomenon for themselves after the probation officer had pointed it out. We would have had an even more difficult task convincing the police, the volunteer and the secure unit staff that something had inhibited their capacity to think. For example in the case of the police, what prevented a five-minute computer check that would have told them that they had a rapist and not a crank? However, the suggestion that they had unwittingly become embroiled in a re-enactment of an unconscious drama would doubtless have met with great resistance.

If our clients seem manipulative or as though they are deliberately trying to "sabotage" our work, it is a facet of *their problem* that we are witnessing and which would be useful to try and understand as an aid to case management. If "blame" is to be pursued—for the professionals' unwanted acts and feelings—it is not the offender's conscious that is to blame but his unconscious internal world. The "sabotaging" effect, which we may think of in terms of pressure to take on the assigned role, is rarely obvious from the perspective of the "actors", as in the example. If, however, it can be assumed that pressure will always be present from the beginning then it allows the opportunity to observe the effect dynamically and thoughts and feelings monitored in relation to the subject. This is similar to, but in some ways more difficult than, the understanding of the transference and counter-transference in the psychoanalytic treatment setting. It does not have the advantage of a regular sustained contact with the patient to elicit gradually the nature of projections and instead requires each involved practitioner to think independently and then in combination with others.

The internal world

The example I have given is one in which a glimpse of the internal world drama is made manifest first through the offences and then again reproduced in the external network. If we think of the client as the "powerless" child whose internal experience is that of a sadistic mother who keeps him there to hurt him, then we have a view of somebody who, when with the female worker or the volunteer, feels powerless against their sadism as he sees it.

The network

It is common sense and obvious good practice that professionals should liaise where appropriate, particularly in high risk cases. However, as I have said, people do not always communicate and work together even when it seems essential. What was it that inhibited the workers saying to each other "let's talk, something is going wrong here"?

Professionals come onto the scene piecemeal and different disciplines have little common purpose. They may all agree that offending is undesirable but after that they may have widely differing objectives, which may inhibit liaison when this is indicated. Welldon (1994, p.470) draws our attention to the differences between the interests of law and psychiatry and also between forensic psychotherapy in general and the criminal justice system. Even within the relatively new hybrid of forensic psychotherapy there will be differing objectives between some of its component disciplines. The Forensic psychiatrist may have a duty to a court while the forensic psychotherapist will have a duty to his patient; sometimes both these roles exist in one person. In general professionals working in parallel may need to liaise frequently but I have addressed in my example how difficulties can occur in this apparently ordinary situation. I conclude therefore that the concept of "professional network" as it is commonly used may just be another "suspect" in the search for an explanation of the phenomena that I have been describing.

Perhaps the term "offender-network" could be used to describe the troupe of potential actors for the pre-assigned roles which were cast within the internal world of the offender. This would be a "network" owned and controlled by the offender with a common purpose to make the external world conform to the internal world. The offence-preview referred to earlier suggests something hopeful but this will be obscured as it is often hidden by the main plot as well as by confusing sub-plots. Ideally, from the "hopeful" perspective the "offender-network" would never recruit any actual players. In other words, as each professional becomes involved they immediately begin the process of identifying the allotted role(s) and resisting it.

Some preliminary thoughts arising from consultancy work in prisons

The view of an outsider

In his own very forthright and human style, Sir David (now Lord) Ramsbotham, in his excellent book *Prison Gate* (Free Press 2003), saw bureaucracy, mismanagement and a reluctance to reform as responsible for keeping Britain's prisons in the dark ages. I would add one more "offender" to his list: the failure to recognize unconscious processes.

I have said above that to manage an offender in the community, a network of professionals has to struggle to retain independent thought and not comply with the offender's script; this is particularly essential in the case of a high risk offender if harm to self or others is to be avoided. If the "plot" can be detected then the professional may be able to write the script.

I would view the "community" of the prison as presenting more complex issues for the objectives of punishment, security, safety, welfare and rehabilitation and, if available, treatment. Unlike the loose group of professionals in the community setting that comes together in response to the individual, the "network" in the prison pre-exists the prisoner's arrival. It is convinced that it already knows the "plot" and has already decided how the drama will be produced and directed.

The route to a prison is via the court where the offender has, albeit briefly, been the centre of attention. In the court he is a man with a name and a history surrounded by judges, barristers, solicitors, probation officers, policemen, ushers, clerks and the public gallery. This is the one opportunity for making sense of his offence and addressing it appropriately. Along with all the conscious motives for the offence there will also be the unconscious meaning of the offence and the equally unconscious wish for it to be understood. It would follow that a response based on such understanding, depending on how embedded is the need for repetition of offending, would reduce and obviate the requirement for further offending. Self evidently an impossible task for a court, but one which nevertheless it does sometimes attempt to understand through court reports from various professionals.

If a prison sentence is the outcome then individuality is immediately replaced with a prison number. He becomes the subject of a system that is not designed to take into account personality or emotional needs. He has gone from being the "special" individual in the court to the unspecial member of a very large group differentiated largely by numbers and wing location, with some additional categorizations such as *vulnerable* or *in need of special diet, segregation* or *treatment for substance abuse*. All his physical needs as well as those of society in relation to him are treated as functions.

From the prison service website:

> Her Majesty's Prison Service serves the public by keeping in custody those committed by the courts. Our duty is to look after them with humanity and help them lead law-abiding and useful lives in custody and after release:
>
> - holding prisoners securely;
> - reducing the risk of prisoners re-offending;
> - providing safe and well-ordered establishments in which we treat prisoners humanely, decently and lawfully.

Within the "closed" system of the prison the "network" of prison officers, governors, discipline, administrative staff, psychiatrists,

GPs, probation officers, cooks, maintenance, instructors, psychologists, nurses, psychiatric nurses, teachers, priests, chaplains, is "preformed" and "ready" for the arrival of each prisoner. It is designed to control, lock up, feed, discipline, transport, educate, sometimes treat, reform, care for, assess, and process. It assumes, in effect, an empty slate upon which to administer the various functions. While it aims to treat "humanely" this does not mean in practice "as a whole human being". All the component parts of the prisoner have been separately catered for and are separately addressed.

Structurally[3] it is built in to a prison to ignore each "inmate's" developmental and life history and any of the pain, anguish, rage, violence or perversion that brought him to this juncture. Every function of the internal world of the prison is directed at the present. Healthcare staff report that inmates often arrive without any "history" and as if they began their existence in the prison. Each event and each behaviour is dealt with as having arisen in the present.

Co-ordination and communication is limited between and within professions, whether security or welfare. Each function might be considered as being applied in isolation from all other functions as though that is *all* the inmate requires. I have sometimes thought during my work that each inmate exists separately in the minds of each profession or discipline such that multiples of the inmate exist within the prison according to the number of functions being applied. The separateness of function and lack of acknowledgement of the value of other professions is described well by Dr Robert Hinshelwood (2004: pp. 121–122) when he refers to "the asserted value of strength and toughness (of the officers) manifested in the ordered rituals of locking and controlling" and the way that "caring attitudes (of the welfare staff, nurses, doctors, psychotherapists, visitors) were exaggerated as over trusting, acquiescing and foolishly gullible". The caring staff for their part view the officers as obstructive and as a resistance to be overcome in order to perform their function.

There are well known symbols of this obstruction: two examples relate to provision and removal of keys and the sudden movement of prisoners such that they cannot be located by caring staff. Rivalrous, envious, denigrating and dismissive attitudes all come into play. When collaboration is required, usually to manage a particular situation, there may be an atmosphere of co-operation and communication but decisions and understandings are frequently later undermined. Prison staff may baulk at these notions and of course it is the wish of the majority to do their jobs professionally and humanely. However, from discussions with prison staff themselves, they will frequently be critical of other sections while also saying how badly they themselves feel treated by the "system" and made to feel inhuman or forgotten.

Visitors to prisons know of the system and may promise themselves they will not become part of it but despite that they are quickly made to comply with the regime. Many social workers, probation officers, lawyers and psychiatrists appear at prison gate reception to be told their client has been moved to another prison overnight ("ghosted"); or cannot be seen as he is "in his woodwork class", "at lunch", "does not wish to see you". All this despite elaborate prior arrangement with the prison on endlessly re-routing automatic telephone redirection systems: visitors discover that their credentials are only worth what the prison deems them to be worth at any given moment.

New staff to a prison will become acutely and immediately aware of the enhanced lack of communication, hostility to change and will quickly experience the undermining behaviour. Two healthcare managers in London prisons attempted to make changes within their own department, departing three and four months later respectively when they realized the impossibility of their task. Many prison governors do not survive in post for very long when perhaps initial optimism and hope has quickly faded.

Discussion

People who commit crimes create fear, anxiety and excitement in us to varying degrees. High profile prisoners in particular attract much excitement, the paparazzi at court rooms and police stations being a familiar sight on television news. Depending on the nature of the crime, they may attract loathing, hatred and vilification, dismissal, curiosity, anger, sympathy or even admiration at the audacity of the offence.

It seems to be a phenomenon that once the subject has been

imprisoned they are largely forgotten. The excitement, fear and anxiety in the public and the professional interest of those at the time of the court hearing dissipate. It is as though something has been satisfied or calmed. If, however, we understood the stimulus in others to be created by the unconscious impact of the unconscious meaning of the offence (projections) then we have a tentative glimpse of the internal world of the inmate-to-be where instead of *violence* we may substitute *fear*; instead of a *brash toughness* we may substitute *anxiety* and instead of a *bland dullness* we may substitute *excitement* that has been generated through early sexualization of aggression at the hands of others. Low profile criminals are not exempt from this process and the terms "petty offender" or "small time crook" leading to summary trial without any attempt to understand the meaning of the actions suggest a dismissive and neglectful attitude perhaps reflecting an internal world where worthlessness, self denigration and a sense of ineffectual smallness prevail.

On visiting a prison for the first time a professional may immediately become aware of the palpable *lack* of excitement, fear and anxiety. Yet that these states continue to exist somewhere may be exemplified by the release of projections at the Johnny Cash concert in San Quentin prison:

> Johnny Cash thanked the warden for allowing the concert, eliciting the expected jeers countered with "aw you don't mean that" which was met with cheers; later on, a song "I shot a man in Reno just to watch him die" produced more cheers and much excitement.

Denigration of the harsh and cruel authority and the apparent lack of capacity for warm feelings of appreciation, with a projected denigration of the weakness and softness as Hinshelwood describes (2004: p. 122) into the warden for providing them with their hero. The identification with inhuman and harsh brutality indicated by the cheers was perhaps also experienced as an interpretation . . . a recognition of inhumanity . . . "At last somebody really understands that it's not anger or pleasure or hatred . . . but 'simply' 'I'll watch him die in the same way somebody watched me (psychically) die' and I'll have no feelings in the way they appeared not to have."

Prison staff are no different from other humans and subject to the same feelings of anxiety, fear and excitement. They will fear violence and be made to feel anxious by unpredictable "madness" such as an inmate attempting suicide or "kicking off" in an inexplicable rage. They attempt to control their fear and anxiety through rituals and through a macho camaraderie. I was told about an inmate who was in a straitjacket in a small special cell, *within a cell*, who had been shouting angrily for some hours. He was on an "eight man lock down" which meant that the psychiatrist was not allowed in to administer medication before eight officers in helmets, riot gear and shields preceded him. They rushed into the cell to pin the already powerless inmate down. The psychiatrist somehow had to try and access his patient in an area designed to accommodate three people.

Caring and healthcare staff are also not immune and divisions may exist between *in*-patient and *out*-patient units that may sometimes be understood as vulnerable at-risk inmates creating anxiety that has become intolerable.

The prison structure and regime inherently supports the continuance of splits and what I have described as the application of functions in isolation and in so doing hopes to contain that which would arouse anxiety and threaten the stability of the prison. It does not do this deliberately but as a social system defending itself against anxiety in much the same way as Isobel Menzies-Lyth describes in her seminal paper (1959; 1988) on the study of a teaching hospital. In so doing it replicates the life histories and internal worlds of the inhabitants of the prison who, each through their development, will have experienced themselves as a function. It might have been as the child to be scapegoated and punished to protect another or perhaps as the child who attempted to isolate his mind from the sexual abuse of his body.

In this way through the perennial failure to acknowledge the unconscious impact of its inmates the prison structure has been *pre-enlisted* to enact in some way the internal world drama of each prisoner.

Within the prison the inmates too need to reinforce their system of social defences against their own perpetual internal anxiety and excitement. If or when lesions appear in the prison structure from time to time to threaten their defence, they may act in some way to restore the equilibrium. Riots and hunger strikes are means by which order can be re-established to provoke the readjustment they require for harsher control and security. In this way the inmate is not exposed to the threat of change through applying constant unconscious pressure on the prison staff to behave as (part) objects familiar to their internal worlds. Poor conditions, neglect, overcrowding, corruption, and violence only serve to reinforce.

Endnote

I have made some broad statements to convey some provisional thoughts, understanding and impressions derived from my contact with prisons in different contexts over 31 years.

It is a preliminary psychoanalytical-structural view and does not intend criticism of much important and valuable work that is carried out by individuals and teams working in prisons, some of which I have had the privilege to witness. Such work, however, continues to be in an environment that opposes integrated thinking and linking that would allow prisoners to be treated as whole human beings and not a collection of fragments to be treated in isolation.

Organizational change can only really be possible when authorized by central government. One such welcome change in recent years has been the gradual introduction of the NHS into prisons, initially with provision of In-Reach "community" mental health teams and primary care services. Perhaps because they have no history in prisons and the staff have experience of working in the community they have begun to make a positive impact after 6 years. They are making their transition from that of imposed outsiders to integrated but essentially independent thinking groups able to maintain an overview. For those with which I have worked I have been made aware that they are effective in carrying out their task in a human way.

Notes

1. The first section of this chapter is a revision of "The Interdisciplinary Network and the Internal World of the Offender" published in C. Cordess & M. Cox (Eds.) (1996), *Forensic Psychotherapy*, Vol. 2. London: Jessica Kingsley.
2. The case predates requirements relating to schedule 1 offenders.
3. This is not to deny, of course, that many professionals in a prison respond individually to inmates in both a professional and a human way.

REFERENCES

Aitkenhead, D. (2006). *Saturday Guardian*, Family section (25.02.06).

Alvarez, A. (1992). *Live Company: Psychoanalytic Psychotherapy with Autistic, Borderline, Deprived and Abused Children*. London & New York: Tavistock/Routledge

Alvarez, A. (1996). Addressing the Element of Deficit in Children With Autism: Psychotherapy Which is Both Psychoanalytically and Developmentally Informed. *Clinical Child Psychology and Psychiatry*, *1*(4): 525–537.

Alvarez, A. (1997). Projective Identification as a Communication: Its Grammar in Borderline Psychotic Children. *Psychoanalytic Dialogue*, *7*(6): 753–768.

American Psychiatric Association (1997). *Diagnostic and Statistical Manual of Mental Disorders* (4th Edn.). Washington, DC: APA.

American Psychiatric Association (2000). *The Diagnostic and Statistical Manual of Mental Disorders* (4th Edn.), Text Revision (DSM IV-TR). Washington DC: APA.

Andersen, H. C. (1857). *The Emperor's New Clothes*. London: Harcourt (1998).

Antebi, D. (2003). Pathways of Risk: The Past, the Present, and the Unconscious. In: R. Doctor (Ed.), *Dangerous Patients: A Psychodynamic Approach to Risk Assessment and Management*, pp. 7–19. London: Karnac Books.

Balint, M. (1968). The Various Forms of Therapeutic Regression. In M. Balint, *The Basic Fault: Therapeutic Aspects of Regression*. London: Routledge.

Bentovim, A. (1993). Why do Adults Sexually Abuse Children? *British Medical Journal, 307*: 144–145.

Bentovim, A., & Davenport, M. (1992). Resolving the Trauma Organised System of Sexual Abuse by Confronting the Abuser. *Journal of Family Therapy, 14*: 29–50.

Berkowitz, R., Dermen, S., Gamble, D., Hakeem, A., Minne, C., & Woods, J. (2002). Transsexuals Need Therapy Not Surgery. Letter to *The Daily Telegraph*, 15th July 2002.

Bion, W. R. (1957). The Differentiation of Psychotic from Non-Psychotic Personalities. *International Journal of Psychoanalysis, 36*: 266–275.

Bion, W. R. (1959). Attacks on Linking. *International Journal of Psychoanalysis, 40*: 308–315.

Bion, W. R. (1962a). A Theory of Thinking, *International Journal of Psychoanalysis, 43*: 306–310.

Bion, W. R. (1962b). *Learning from Experience*. London: Heinemann. [Reprinted London: Karnac Books, 1984.]

Blos, P. (1967). The Second Individuation Process of Adolescence. *Psychoanalytic Study of the Child, 22*: 162–186.

Bollas, C. (2003). Confidentiality and Professionalism in Psychoanalysis. *British Journal of Psychotherapy, 20*(2): 157–176.

Bollas, C., & Sundelson, D. (1995). *The New Informants: Betrayal of Confidentiality in Psychoanalysis and Psychotherapy*. London: Karnac Books.

Bowlby, J. (1944). Forty Four Juvenile Thieves: Their Characters and Home Life. *International Journal of Psychoanalysis, 25*: 19–52.

Bowlby, J. (1973). *Attachment and Loss, Vol. 2, Separation*, London: Hogarth Press.

Bowlby, J. (1980). *Attachment and Loss, Vol. 3, Loss*, London: Hogarth Press.

Brenman, E. (2003). Foreword in *The Sadomasochistic Perversion* by F. De Massi. London: Karnac.

Britton, R. (1989). The Missing Link: Parental Sexuality in the Oedipus Complex. In J. Steiner (Ed.), *The Oedipus Complex Today: Clinical Implications*. London: Karnac Books.

Britton, R., Feldman, M., & O'Shaughnessy, E. (1989). *The Oedipus Complex Today: Clinical Implications*, John Steiner (Ed.). London: Karnac Books.

Buchanan, A. (1999). Risk and Dangerousness. *Psychological Medicine, 29*: 465–473.

Burou, G. (1974). Quoted in *Titne*, 21st January, p. 64.

Buxbaum, E. (1970). Aggression and the Function of the Group in Adolescence. In *Troubled Children in a Troubled World*, New York: International Universities Press.

Campbell, D. (1994). Breaching the Shame Shield: Thoughts on the Assessment of Adolescent Child Sexual Abusers. *Journal of Child Psychotherapy, 20*(3): 309–326.

Caper, R. (1999). *A Mind of One's Own*. London and New York: Routledge.

Carnes, P. J. (2000). Toward the DSM-V: How Science and Personal Reality Meet. *Sexual Addiction and Compulsivity, 7*: 157–160.

Carnes, P. J., Delmonico, D. L., & Griffin, E. J. (2001). *In the Shadows of the Net: Breaking Free from Compulsive Online Sexual Behaviour*. Center City, NH: Hazledon Foundation Press.

Chasseguet-Smirgel, J. (1981). Loss of Reality in the Perversions – with Special Reference to Fetishism. *Journal of the American Psychoanalytic Association, 29*: 511–534.

Chasseguet-Smirgel, J. (1985). *Creativity and Perversion*. London: Free Association Books. clickz.com/stats/web-worldwide/ (visited 7.5.06).

Cooper, A. (1997). The Internet and Sexuality: Into the New Millennium. *Journal of Sex Education and Therapy, 22*: 5–6.

Cooper, A. (Ed.) (2002). *Sex and the Internet*. New York: Brunner Routledge.

Cooper, A., & Griffin-Shelley, E. (2002). Introduction. The Internet: The Next Sexual Revolution. In A. Cooper (Ed.) (2002). *Sex and the Internet*. New York: Brunner Routledge.

Cooper, A., Delmonico, D., & Burg, R. (2000). Cybersex Users and Abusers: New Findings and Implications. *Sexual Addiction and Compulsivity: Journal of Treatment and Prevention, 1–2*: 5–30.

Cooper, A., McLoughlin, I. P., & Campbell, K. M. (2000). Sexuality in Cyberspace: Update for the 21st Century. *CyberPsychology and Behaviour, 3*(4): 521–536.

Cooper, A., Scherer, C., Boies, S. C., & Gordon, B. (1999). Sexuality on the Internet: From Sexual Exploration to Pathological Expression. *Professional Psychology: Research and Practice, 30*(2): 154–164.

Cordess, C. & Cox, M. (Eds.) (1996). *Forensic Psychotherapy: Crime, Psychodynamics and the Offender Patient*. London: Jessica Kingsley Publishers.

Cox, M. (1994). Manipulation. *Journal of Forensic Psychiatry, 5*(1): 9–13.

Davies, R. (1996). The Inter-disciplinary Network and the Internal World of the Offender. In C. Cordess, & M. Cox (Eds.), *Forensic Psychotherapy: Crime, Psychodynamics and the Offender Patient. Vol. II: Mainly Practice*. London: Jessica Kingsley.

Delmonico, D. L., Griffin, E., & Carnes, P. J. (2002). Treating Online Compulsive Sexual Behaviour: When Cybersex is the Drug of Choice. In A. Cooper (Ed.) (2002). *Sex and the Internet*. New York: Brunner Routledge.

Di Ceglie, G. (1995). From the Couple to the Marital Relationship. In *Intrusiveness and Intimacy in the Couple*. S. Ruszczynski & J. Fisher (Eds.). London: Karnac Books.

Dicks, H. V. (1970). *Fifty Years of the Tavistock Clinic*. London: Routledge and Kegan Paul.

Doctor, R. (2003). *Dangerous Patients: A Psychodynamic Approach to Risk Assessment and Management*, pp. 7–19. London: Karnac Books.

Edgcumbe, R. (1976). The Development of Aggressiveness in Children. *Nursing Times*, 1st April (RCN Supplement): vii–xv.

Edgcumbe, R. (1988). Formulation of interpretations in clinical work with adolescents. Unpublished paper given at the Institute of Psycho-analysis, London, October.

Edgcumbe, R., & Burgner, M. (1975). The Phallic Narcissistic Phase: A Differentiation Between Pre-Oedipal and Oedipal Aspects of Phallic Development. *Psychoanalytic Study of the Child, 30*: 161–180 (New York: International Universities Press).

European Court of Human Rights (2002). *Case of Christine Goodwin v. The United Kingdom* (Application no. 28957195). Judgment Strasbourg, 11 July 2002.

Farrington, D. P. (2003). Advancing Knowledge about the Early Prevention of Adult Anti-social Behaviour. In: Farrington, D. P. and Coid, J. W. (Eds), *Early Prevention of Adult Antisocial Behaviour*. Cambridge: Cambridge University Press.

Feldman, M. (2000). Some Views on the Manifestation of the Death Instinct in Clinical Work. *International Journal of Psychoanalysis, 81*: 53–65.

Fenichel, O. (1945). Neurotic Acting Out. *Psychoanalytic Review, 32*: 197–206.

Ferree, M. C. (2003). Women and the Web: Cybersex Activity and Implications. *Sexual and Relationship Therapy, 18*(3): 385–393.

Fonagy, P. (2003). Towards a Developmental Understanding of Violence. *British Journal of Psychiatry, 183*: 190–192.

Fonagy, P., & Target, M. (1995). Understanding the Violent Patient: The Use of the Body and the Role of the Father. *International Journal of Psychoanalysis, 76*: 487–501.

Fonagy, P., & Target, M. (1996). A Contemporary Psychoanalytical Perspective: Psychodynamic Developmental Therapy. In E. Hibbs & P. Jensen (Eds.), *Psychosocial Treatments for Child and Adolescent Disorders*. Washington, DC: American Psychological Association.

Fonagy, P., Gergely, G., Jurist, E. L., & Target, M. (2002). *Affect Regulation, Mentalisation and the Development of the Self*. New York: Other Press.

Fraiberg, S. (1982). Pathological Defences in Infancy. *Psychoanalytic Quarterly, 51*: 612–635.

Freud, A. (1936/1942). *The Ego and the Mechanisms of Defence*. London: Hogarth Press.

Freud, A. (1949). Aggression in Relation to Emotional Development: Normal and Pathological. *Psychoanalytic Study of the Child, 3/4*: 37–42. New York: International Universities Press.

Freud, A. (1958). Adolescence. *Psychoanalytic Study of the Child, 13*: 255–278 (New York: International Universities Press).

Freud, A. (1965). *Normality and Pathology in Childhood*, London: Hogarth.

Freud, A. (1968). Difficulties in the Path of Psychoanalysis: A Confrontation of Past With Present Viewpoints. In *The Writings of Anna Freud Vol. VII 1966–1970: Problems of Psychoanalytic Training, Diagnosis, and the Technique of Therapy*. New York: International Universities Press, 1971.

Freud, A. (1972). Comments on Aggression. In *Psychoanalytic Psychology of Normal Development*. London: Hogarth Press (1982).

Freud, A. (1980). *Normality and Pathology in Childhood: Assessments of Development*. London: Hogarth Press.

Freud, S. (1896). *Further Remarks of the Neuro-Psychoses of Defence, Standard Edition 3*. London: Hogarth Press, p. 159.

Freud, S. (1905). *Three Essays on Sexuality, Standard Edition 7*. London: Hogarth Press.

Freud, S. (1914). *Remembering, Repeating and Working-through* (Further Recommendations on the Technique of Psycho-analysis, II), *Standard Edition 12*. London: Hogarth Press.

Freud, S. (1916–1917). Introductory Lectures on Psycho-Analysis. Ch. XXIII *The Paths to the Formation of Symptoms, Standard Editions 15–16*. London: Hogarth Press.

Freud, S. (1919). *A Child is Being Beaten, Standard Edition 17*. London: Hogarth Press.

Freud, S. (1920). *Beyond the Pleasure Principle, Standard Edition 18*. London: Hogarth Press.

Freud, S. (1923). *The Ego and the Id, Standard Edition 19*. London: Hogarth Press.

Freud, S. (1926). *Inhibitions, Symptoms and Anxiety, Standard Edition 20*. London: Hogarth Press.

Freud, S. (1927). *Fetishism, Standard Edition 21*. London: Hogarth Press.

Freud, S. (1940). *Splitting of the Ego in the Process of Defence, Standard Edition 23*. London: Hogarth Press.

Freud, S., & Breuer, J. (1895). *Studies on Hysteria, Standard Edition 20*. London: Hogarth Press.

Furman, E. (1992). *Toddlers and Their Mothers. A Study in Early Personality Development*, Madison, CT: International Universities Press.

Gabbard, G. O. (2001). Cyberpassion: E-rotic Transference on the Internet. *Psychoanalytic Quarterley, LXX*: 719–737.

General Medical Council (2004). *Confidentiality: Protecting and Providing Information*. London: GMC Publications.

Gilligan, J. (2000). *Violence: Reflections on our Deadliest Epidemic*. London: Jessica Kingsley Publishers.

Glasser, M. (1964). Aggression and Sadism in the Perversions. In I. Rosen (Ed.), *Sexual Deviation*. Oxford: Oxford University Press, pp. 279–300.

Glasser, M. (1979). Some Aspects of the Role of Aggression in the Perversions. In: I. Rosen (Ed.), *Sexual Deviation* (2nd edn.). Oxford: Oxford University Press.

Glasser, M. (1979a). Some Aspects of the Role of Aggression in the Perversions. In I. Rosen (Ed.), *Sexual Deviation* (2nd Edn.). Oxford, New York, Toronto: Oxford University Press.

Glasser, M. (1979b). From the Analysis of a Transvestite. *International Review of Psycho-Analysis, 6*: 163.

Glasser, M. (1985). "The Weak Spot": Some Observations on Male Homosexuality. *International Journal of Psychoanalysis, 66*: 405–414.

Glasser, M. (1988). Psychodynamic Aspects of Paedophilia, *Psychoanalytic Psychotherapy 3*(2): 121–135.

Glasser, M. (1996). Aggression and Sadism in the Perversions. In I. Rosen, (Ed.), *Sexual Deviation* (3rd Edn). Oxford: Oxford University Press.

Glasser, M. (1998). On Violence: A Preliminary Communication. *International Journal of Psychoanalysis, 79*: 887–902.

Glover, E. (1933). The Relation of Perversion-Formation to the Development of Reality Sense. *International Journal of Psycho-Analysis, 14*: 4.

Glover, E. (1956). *The Early Development of Mind*. London: Imago Publishing.

Glover, E. (1960). *The Roots of Crime*. London: Imago Publishing.

Green, A. (1986). Negation and Contradiction (Chapter 10). In: *Private Madness*. London: Maresfield Press.

Greenfield, D. N. (1999). Psychological Characteristics of Compulsive Internet Use: A Preliminary Analysis. *CyberPsychology and Behaviour, 2*(5): 403–412.

Greenfield, D. N., & Davis, R. A. (2002). Lost in Cyberspace: The Web@Work. *CyberPsychology and Behaviour, 5*(4): 347–353.

Greenfield, D. N., & Orzak, M. (2002). The Electronic Bedroom: Clinical Assessment of Online Sexual Problems and Internet-Enabled Sexual Behaviour. In A. Cooper (Ed.). *Sex and the Internet*. New York: Brunner Routledge.

Griffen-Shelly, E. (2003). The Internet and Sexuality: A Literature Review – 1983–2002. *Sexual and Relationship Therapy, 18*(3): 355–370.

Hale, R. (2003). Setting the Scene 1: From Common Law to Statute Law. *British Journal of Psychotherapy, 20*(2): pp. 135–139.

Hamilton, D. (2002). Transvestite Prejudice. Letter in response, *The Daily Telegraph* 20th July 2002.

Hari, J. (2004). Paedophiles Need More Understanding. *The Independent*, 27th October.

Harry Benjamin International Gender Dysphoria Association (2001). *The Standards of Care for Gender Identity Disorders*. Sixth Version. Dusseldorf: Symposion Publishing.

Hartnup, T. (1999). The Therapeutic Setting. In A. Horne & M. Lanyado (Eds.), *The Handbook of Child and Adolescent Psychotherapy*. London: Routledge.

Hartocollis, P. (2001). *Mankind's Oedipal Destiny*. Madison, CT: International Universities Press.

Heimann, P., & Valenstein, A. (1972). The Psychoanalytical Concept of Aggression: An Integrated Summary. *International Journal of Psycho-Analysis, 53*: 31–35.

Hinshelwood, R. D. (2004). *Suffering Insanity*. London: Brunner Routledge.

Hoffer, W. (1949). Mouth, Hand, and Ego-integration. *Psychoanalytic Study of the Child, 3/4*: 49–56 (New York: International Universities Press).

Horne, A. (1999). Sexual Abuse and Sexual Abusing in Childhood and Adolescence. In M. Lanyado & A. Horne (Eds.), *The Handbook of Child and Adolescent Psychotherapy: Psychoanalytic Perspectives*. London: Routledge.

Hurry, A. (1998). Psychoanalysis and Developmental Therapy. In A. Hurry (Ed.), *Psychoanalysis and Developmental Therapy*. London: Karnac.

Hyatt Williams, A. (1995). Murderousness in Relation to Psychotic Breakdown (Madness). In J. Ellwood (Ed.) *Psychosis: Understanding and Treatment*. London and Bristol/Pennsylvania: Jessica Kingsley.

Hyatt Williams, A. (1998). *Cruelty, Violence and Murder*. London: Jason Aronson.

Johns, M. (2002). Identification and Dis-identification in the Development of Sexual Identity. In J. Trowell & A. Etchegoyen (Eds.), *The Importance of Fathers*. London: Brunner Routledge, pp. 186–202.

Jurgen, F., Shepherd, A., & Ferguson, B. G. (2002). What Services are Available for the Treatment of Transsexuals in Great Britain? *Psychiatric Bulletin: The Journal of Psychiatric Practice. 26*: 6.

Khan, M. (1973). The Concept of Cumulative Trauma. *Psychoanalytic Study of the Child, 18*: 286–306 (New York: International Universities Press).

King's Fund (2003). *London's State of Mind: King's Fund Mental Health Inquiry 2003*. London: King's Fund Publications.

Klein, M. (1946). Notes on Some Schizoid Mechanisms. In: M. Klein, P. Heimann, S. Isaacs, & J. Riviere (Eds.) *Developments in Psycho-Analysis*. London: Hogarth Press, 1952. [Reprinted London: Karnac Books, 1989.]

Kolvin, I., & Trowell, J. (1996). Child Sexual Abuse. In I. Rosen (Ed.), *Sexual Deviation* (3rd Edn). Oxford: Oxford University Press.

Lanyado, M. and Horne, A. (Eds) (1999). *Handbook of Child and Adolescent Psychotherapy*. London: Routledge.

Lanyado, M., Hodges, J., Bentovim, A. *et al.* (1995). Understanding Boys Who Sexually Abuse Other Children: A Clinical Illustration. *Psychoanalytic Psychotherapy, 9*(3): 231–242.

Laufer, M. (1976). The Central Masturbation Fantasy, the Final Sexual Organization, and Adolescence. *Psychoanalytic Study of the Child, 31*: 297–305.

Laufer, M. E. (1981). The Adolescent's Use of the Body in Object Relationships and in the Transference: A Comparison of Borderline and Narcissistic Modes of Functioning. *Psychoanalytic Study of the Child, 36*: 163–180 (New Haven: Yale University Press).

Leigh, R. (1998). Panel Reports: Perversion. *International Journal of Psychoanalysis, 79*: 1217–1220.

Lewin, R. A., & Schulz, C. (1992). *Losing and Fusing: Borderline Transitional Object and Self Relationships*. Northvale, NJ & London: Jason Aronson.

Limentani, A. (1966). A Re-evaluation of Acting Out in Relation to Working Through. *International Journal of Psychoanalysis, 47*.

Limentani, A. (1989a). *Between Freud and Klein*. London: Free Association Books. [Reprinted London: Karnac Books, 1999.]

Limentani, A. (1989b). The Significance of Transsexualism in Relation to Some Basic Psychoanalytic Concepts. In *Between Freud and Klein: The Psychoanalytic Quest for Knowledge*, Ch. 9, pp. 133–154. London: Free Association Books. [Reprinted London: Karnac Books, 1999.]

Limentani, A. (1989c). Clinical Types of Homosexuality. In *Between Freud and Klein: The Psychoanalytic Quest for Knowledge*, Ch. 7, pp. 102–113. London: Free Association Books. [Reprinted London: Karnac Books, 1999.]

Lloyd-Owen, D. (1997). From Action to Thought: Supervising Mental Health Workers With Forensic Patients. In B. Martindale *et al.* (Eds.), *Supervision and Its Vicissitudes* (EFPP Clinical Monograph Series). London: Karnac Books.

Loewald, H. W. (1960). On the Therapeutic Action of Psychoanalysis. *International Journal of Psychoanalysis, 41*: 16–33.

MacKenna, C. (2003). Ethical Pressures on the Analytic Alliance. In H. M. Solomon & M. Twyman (Eds.), *The Ethical Attitude in Analytic Practice*, pp. 51–64. London: Free Association Books.

McCarthy, B. (1988). Are Incest Victims Hated? *Psychoanalytic Psychotherapy, 3*(2).

McDougall, J. (1972). Primal Scene and Sexual Perversion. *International Journal of Psychoanalysis, 53*: 371–384.

Menzies-Lyth, I. (1988). The Functioning of Social Systems as a Defence Against Anxiety. In *Containing Anxiety in Institutions: Selected Essays*,

Vol. 1. London: Free Association Books. [First published 1959 in *Human Relations* journal.]

Minne, C. (2003). Psychoanalytic Aspects to the Risk Containment of Dangerous Patients Treated in High Security Hospital. In R. Doctor (Ed.), *Dangerous Patients: A Psychodynamic Approach to Risk Assessment and Management*, pp. 61–78. London: Karnac Books.

Monahan, J. (1984). The Prediction of Violent Behaviour: Toward a Second Generation of Theory and Policy. *American Journal of Psychiatry, 141*: 10–15.

Monahan, J. (1993). Limiting Therapist Exposure to Tarasoff Liability: Guidelines for Risk Containment. *American Psychologist, 48*: 242–250.

Money, J., & Elirhard, A. A. (1972). *Man and Woman, Boy and Girl: The Differentiation and Dimorphism of Gender Identity from Conception to Birth.* Baltimore: Johns Hopkins University Press.

Money-Kyrle, R. (1971). The Aim of Psychoanalysis. In D. Meltzer and E. O'Shaughnessy (Eds.), *The Collected Papers of Roger Money-Kyrle.* Perthshire: Clunie Press.

Morgan, D. (2001). Hate as a Pre-requisite for Love (Chapter 7). In: *Love and Hate.* David Mann (Ed.). London: Routledge.

Mullen, P. (1984). Mental Disorder and Dangerousness. *Australian and New Zealand Journal of Psychiatry, 18*: 8–17.

Ogden, T. H. (1966). Reconsidering Three Aspects of Psychoanalytic Technique. *International Journal of Psychoanalysis 77*: 883–899.

Pailthorpe, G. (1932). *Studies in the Psychology of Delinquency* (Medical Research Council Special Report Series). London: Medical Research Council.

Parsons, M., & Dermen, S. (1999). The Violent Child and Adolescent. In M. Lanyado & A. Horne (Eds.), *The Handbook of Child and Adolescent Psychotherapy: Psychoanalytic Perspectives.* London: Routledge.

Quayle, E., & Taylor, M. (2002). Child Pornography and the Internet: Perpetuating a Cycle of Abuse. *Deviant Behaviour, 23*(4): 331–362.

Rado, S. (1933). The Psychoanalysis of Pharmacothymia. *Psychoanalytic Quarterly, 2*: 1–23. Reprinted in D. L. Yalisove (Ed.) (1997). *Essential Papers on Addiction.* New York: New York University Press.

Ramsbotham, D. (2003). *Prison Gate.* UK: The Free Press.

Reed, J. (1997). Risk Assessment and Clinical Risk Management: The Lessons From Recent Inquiries. *British Journal of Psychiatry,* I (suppl. 32): 4–7.

Rey, H. (1987). *Universals of Psychoanalysis.* London: Karnac Books.

Rey, H. (1994). *Universals of Psychoanalysis in the Treatment of Psychotic and Borderline States.* London: Free Association Books.

Rosen, I. (Ed.) (1964), *Sexual Deviation.* Oxford: Oxford University Press.

Rosenfeld, H. A. (1960). On Drug Addiction. *International Journal of*

Psycho-Analysis, 41. Reprinted in *Psychotic States* (1965). London: Hogarth Press/ Karnac Books.

Rosenfeld, H. (1978). Notes on the Psychopathology and Psychoanalytic Treatment of Some Borderline Patients. *International Journal of Psycho-analysis, 59*: 215.

Royal Society of Medicine (2002). *Recent Advances in Gender Dysphoria, Gender Identity Disorder: Towards a Uniform Treatment Approach*. One-day conference organised by the Sexual Health and Reproductive Medicine Section. 16th April 2002.

Ruszczynski, S. (2003). States of Mind in Perversion and Violence. *The Journal of the British Association of Psychotherapists, 41*(2): 87–100.

Ruszczynski, S., & Fisher, J. (1995). *Intrusiveness and Intimacy in the Couple Relationship*. London: Karnac Books.

Sandler, J. (1976). Countertransference and Role-responsiveness. *International Review of Psycho-Analysis, 3*: 43–47.

Saville, E., & Rumney, D. (1992). *"Let Justice be Done!": A History of the ISTD*. London: Institute for the Study and Treatment of Delinquency

Schneider, J. P. (2000). A Qualitative Study of Cybersex Participants: Gender Differences, Recovery Issues and Implications for Therapists. *Sexual Addiction and Compulsivity, 7*: 249–278 (reprinted from the internet: www.jenniferschenider.com/articles/qualitative_cybersex.html, viewed 4.11.03).

Segal, H. (1972). A Delusional System as a Defence Against the Re-emergence of a Catastrophic Situation. *International Journal of Psychoanalysis, 53*: 393–401

Segal, H. (1975a). *An Introduction to the Work of Melanie Klein*. London: Hogarth Press.

Segal, H. (1975b). A Psychoanalytical Approach to the Treatment of Schizophrenia. In M. Lader (Ed.), *Studies of Schizophrenia*. New York: Headley Bros.

Segal, H. (1993). On the Clinical Usefulness of the Concept of the Death Instinct. *International Journal of Psychoanalysis, 74*: 55–61.

Seymour Report (1985). Tavistock and Portman Clinic Review. Report of an Independent Review Group set up by the Minister of State for Health (November 1985). Unpublished.

Shelley, M. (1818). *Frankenstein*. Harmondsworth: Penguin (1994).

Shengold, L. (1989). *Soul Murder: The Effects of Child Abuse and Deprivations*. New Haven, Conn: Yale University Press.

Sher, M. (2003). Ethical Issues for Psychotherapists Working in Organisations. In H. M. Solomon & M. Twyman (Eds.), *The Ethical Attitude in Analytic Practice*, pp. 137–151. London: Free Association Books.

Snowden, P. (1997). Practical Aspects of Clinical Risk Management. *British Journal of Psychiatry, 170*(Suppl. 323): 32–34.

Sohn, L. (1997). Unprovoked Assaults: Making Sense of Apparently Random Violence. In D. Bell (Ed.) *Reason and Passion: A Celebration of the Work of Hanna Segal*. London: Duckworth.

Solomon, H. M. (2003). The Ethical Attitude: A Bridge Between Psychoanalysis and Analytical Psychology. In H. M. Solomon & M. Twyman (Eds.), *The Ethical Attitude in Analytic Practice*. London: Free Association Books.

Sorenson, T., & Hertoft, P. (1980). Sex Modifying Operations on Transsexuals in Denmark in the Period 1950–1977. *Aeta Psychiatrica Scandinavica, 61*: 56–66.

Steiner, J. (1993). *Psychic Retreats*. London and New York: Routledge.

Stern, D. N. (1985). *The Interpersonal World of the Human Infant*. New York: Basic Books.

Stoller, R. J. (1968). *Sex and Gender: The Development of Masculinity and Femininity* London: Karnac Books.

Stoller, R. J. (1975a). *Perversion: The Erotic Form of Hatred*. London: Quartet.

Stoller, R. J. (1975b). *The Transsexual Experiment*. London: Hogarth Press.

Stoller, R. (1976). *Perversion: The Erotic Form of Hatred*. Sussex: The Harvester Press Limited.

Symington, N. (1980). The Response Aroused by the Psychopath. *International Review of Psychoanalysis, 7*.

Taylor, M., & Quayle, E. (2003). *Child Pornography: An Internet Crime*. Hove: Brunner Routledge.

Taylor, P. J., & Estroff, S. E. (2003). Schizophrenia and Violence. In: S. R. Hirsch & D. Weinberger (Eds.), *Schizophrenia*, pp. 591–692. Oxford: Blackwell.

Tepper, M. S., & Owens, A. F. (2002). Access to Pleasure: On Ramp to Specific Information on Disability, Illness, and Changes Throughout the Lifespan. In A. Cooper (Ed.) (2002). *Sex and the Internet*. New York: Brunner Routledge.

Tonnessmann, M. (1980). Adolescent Re-enactment, Trauma and Reconstruction. *Journal of Child Psychotherapy, 6*: 23–44.

Trowell, J., & Etchegoyen, A. (2002). *The Importance of Fathers*, London: Brunner Routledge.

Turpin, A. (2006). Not Tonight, Darling, I'm Online. *Financial Times Magazine*, 1st/2nd April.

Velsen, C. Van (1997). The Victim in the Offender. In H. Van Marle (Ed.), *Challenges in Forensic Psychotherapy*. London: Jessica Kingsley Publishers.

Welldon, E. (1988). *Mother, Madonna, Whore: The Idealisation and Denigration of Motherhood*. London: Free Association Books/ The Guildford Press.

Welldon, E. (1994). Forensic Psychotherapy. In P. Clarkson & M. Pokorny (Eds.), *Handbook of Psychotherapy*. London: Routledge.

Welldon, E. (2001). *Deception as an Artistic Endeavour*. Glover Lecture, unpublished.

Williams, G. (1998). *Internal Landscapes, Foreign Bodies, Eating Disorders and Other Pathologies*. London: Tavistock.

Wilson, P. (1991). Psychotherapy with Adolescents. In J. Holmes (Ed.), *Textbook of Psychotherapy in Psychiatric Practice*. New York: Churchill-Livingstone.

Wilson, P. (1999). Delinquency. In M. Lanyado & A. Horne (Eds.), *The Handbook of Child and Adolescent Psychotherapy – Psychoanalytic Perspectives*. London: Routledge.

Winnicott, D. W. (1947). Hate in the Countertransference. In D. W. Winnicott, *Collected Papers: Through Paediatrics to Psycho-analysis*. London: Hogarth (1978).

Winnicott, D. W. (1950–1955). Aggression in Relation to Emotional Development. In D. W. Winnicott, *Collected Papers: Through Paediatrics to Psycho-analysis*. London: Hogarth (1978).

Winnicott, D. W. (1951). Transitional Objects and Transitional Phenomena. Reprinted in *Through Paediatrics to Psycho-analysis* (1958). London: Hogarth Press.

Winnicott, D. W. (1954). Metapsychological and Clinical Aspects of Regression Within the Psychoanalytic Set-up. In: D. W. Winnicott, *Collected Papers: Through Paediatrics to Psycho-analysis*. London: Tavistock (1958)/Hogarth (1975)/Karnac Books (1991).

Winnicott, D. W. (1956). The Antisocial Tendency. In D. W. Winnicott, *Collected Papers: Through Paediatrics to Psycho-analysis*. London: Tavistock (1958).

Winnicott, D. W. (1959–1964). Classification: Is There a Psychoanalytic Contribution to Psychiatric Classification? In: *The Maturational Processes and the Facilitating Environment*. London: Hogarth Press. [Reprinted London: Karnac Books, 1990.]

Winnicott, D. W. (1962). The Aims of Psycho-analytic Treatment. In *The Maturational Processes and the Facilitating Environment*. London: Hogarth Press (1965).

Winnicott, D. W. (1963a). From Dependence Towards Independence in the Development of the Individual. In D. W. Winnicott, *The Maturational Processes and the Facilitating Environment*. London: Hogarth Press (1979).

Winnicott, D. W. (1963b). The Development of the Capacity for Concern. In D. W. Winnicott, *The Maturational Processes and the Facilitating Environment*. London: Hogarth Press (1979).

Winnicott, D. W. (1963c). Psychotherapy of Character Disorders. In D. W. Winnicott, *The Maturational Processes and the Facilitating Environment*. London: Hogarth Press (1965).

Winnicott, D. W. (1963d). Hospital Care Supplementing Intensive Psychotherapy in Adolescence. In D. W. Winnicott, *The Maturational Processes and the Facilitating Environment*. London: Hogarth Press (1965).

Winnicott, D. W. (1988). *Human Nature*. London: Free Association Books.

Wolf, H. *et al.* (1990). UCH Textbook of Psychiatry. London: Gerald Duckworth.

Wood, H. (2006a). Psychoanalytically-oriented CAT as a First Treatment for Sexual Relationship Problems. In J. Hiller, H. Wood, & W. Bolton (Eds.) *Sex, Mind and Emotion*. London: Karnac.

Wood, H. (2006b). Compulsive Use of Internet Pornography. In J. Hiller, H. Wood, & W. Bolton (Eds.), *Sex, Mind and Emotion*. London: Karnac.

Wood, H., Ramadhan, Z., & Delmar-Morgan, R. (2005). Audit of Portman Clinic Referrals. Unpublished paper.

Woods, J. (2003). *Boys Who Have Abused*. London: Jessica Kingsley Publishers.

Young, R. M. (1996). Primitive Processes on the Internet. Available on www.shef.ac.uk/uni.academic/N-Q/psych/staff/rmyoung.papers (visited 7.3.04).

Young, R. M. (1998). Sexuality and the Internet. Available on http://human-nature.com/rmyoung/papers/pap108h.html (visited 15.4.04).

Young R. M. (2003). Boundaries of Perversion. Available on http://human-nature.com/rmyoung/papers/pap143h.html (visited 4.5.04).

INDEX

Locators shown in *italics* refer to tables.

For Product Safety Concerns and Information please contact our EU representative GPSR@taylorandfrancis.com
Taylor & Francis Verlag GmbH, Kaufingerstraße 24, 80331 München, Germany

www.ingramcontent.com/pod-product-compliance
Ingram Content Group UK Ltd.
Pitfield, Milton Keynes, MK11 3LW, UK
UKHW022204190926
475702UK00003B/196
* 9 7 8 0 3 6 7 3 2 5 3 1 2 *